Dysphagia - New Advances

Edited by Monjur Ahmed

Published in London, United Kingdom

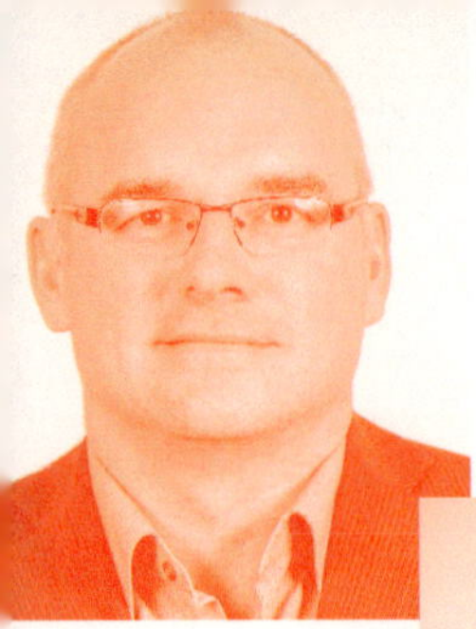
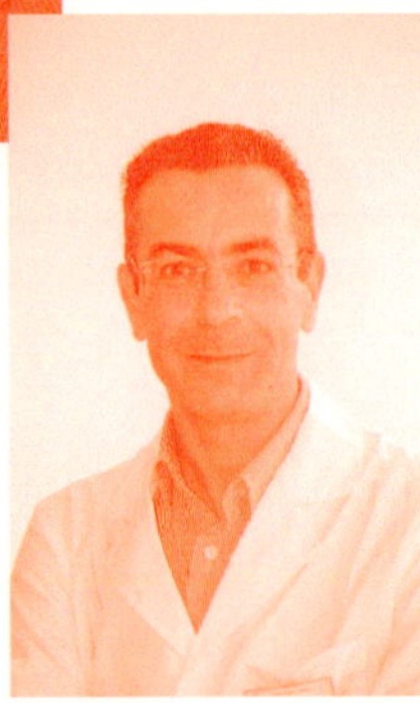
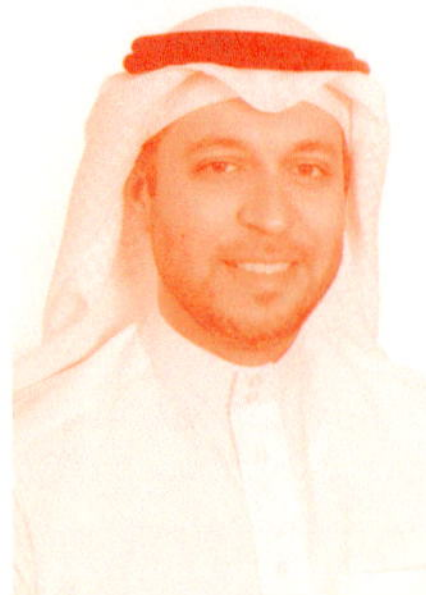
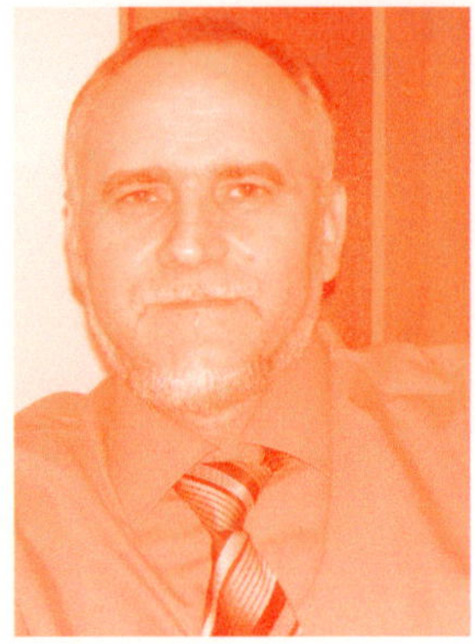
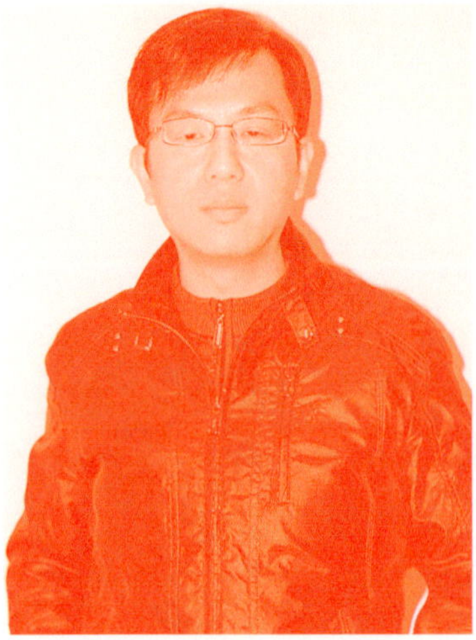
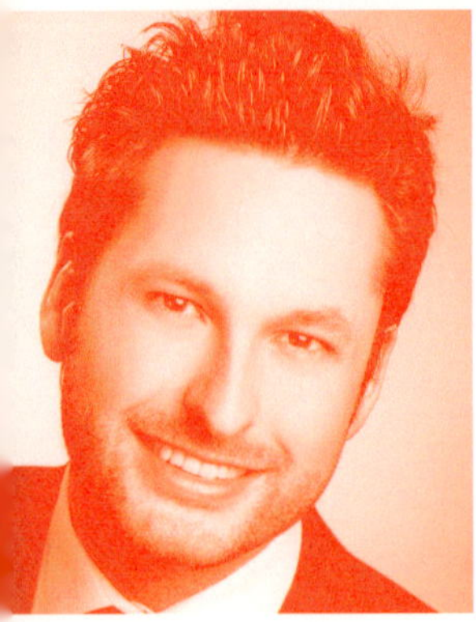
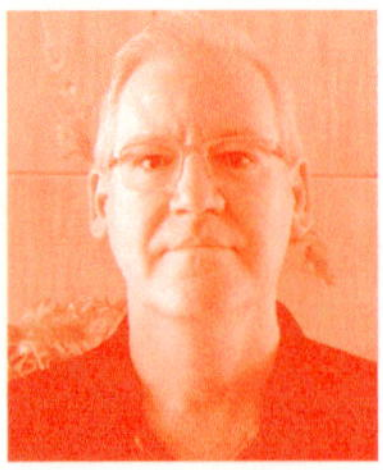

IntechOpen

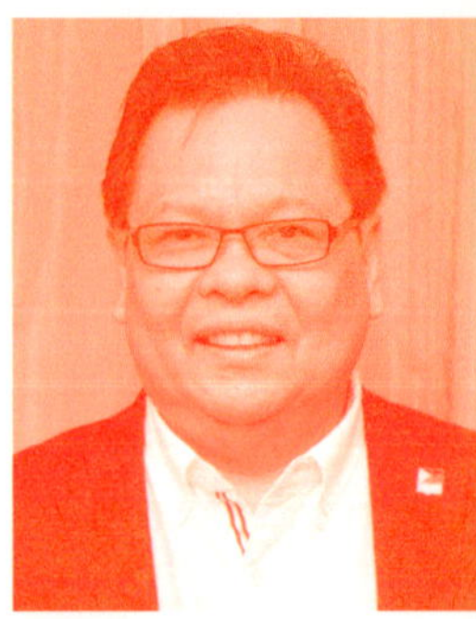
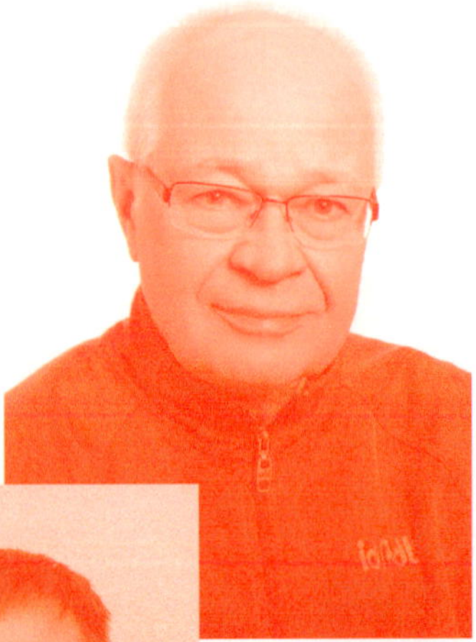
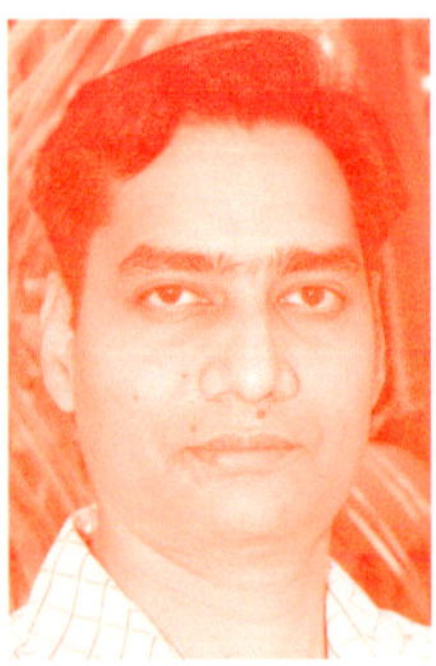
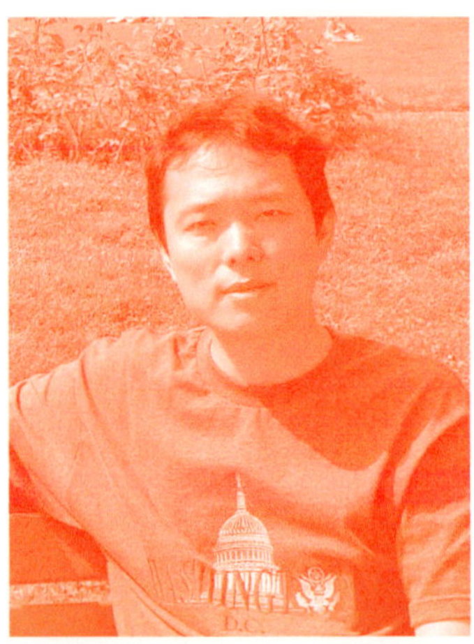
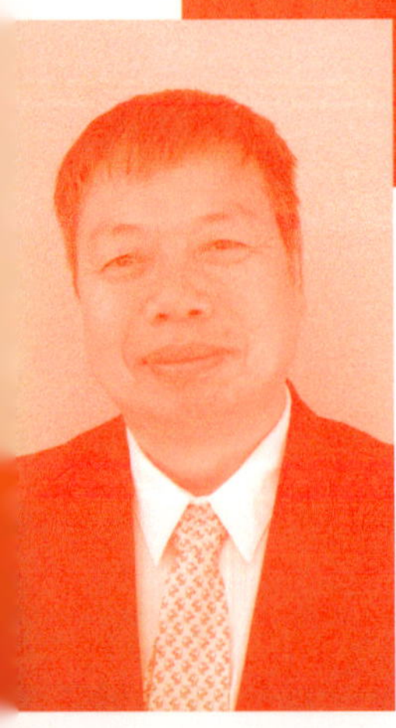
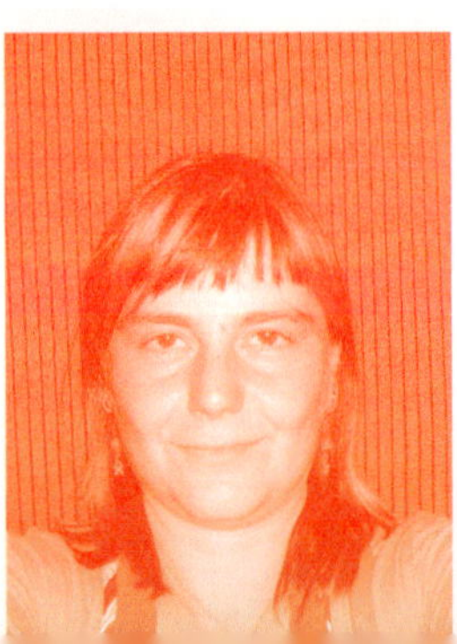

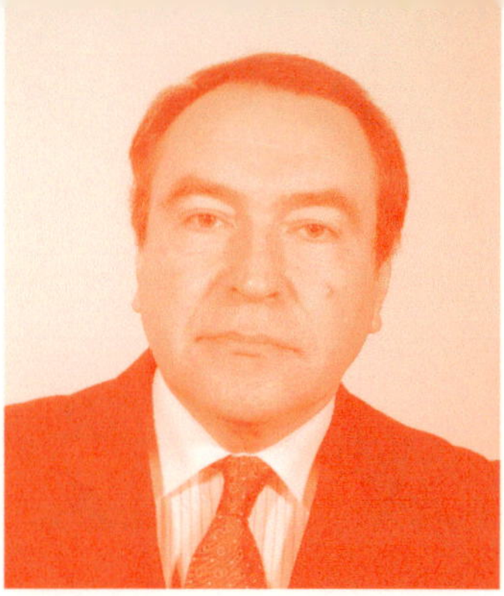
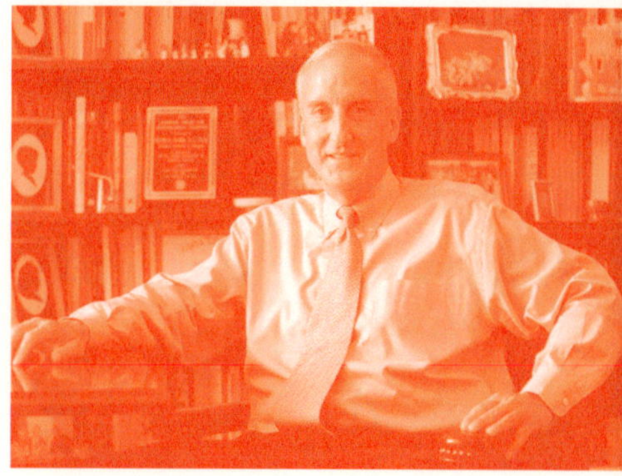
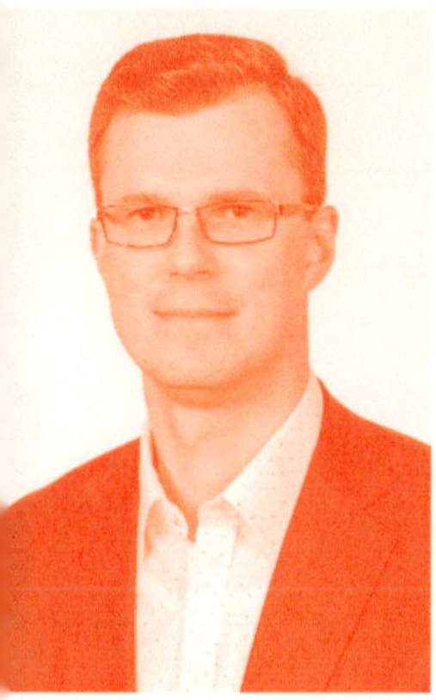
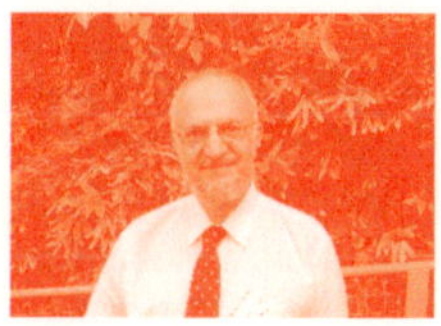
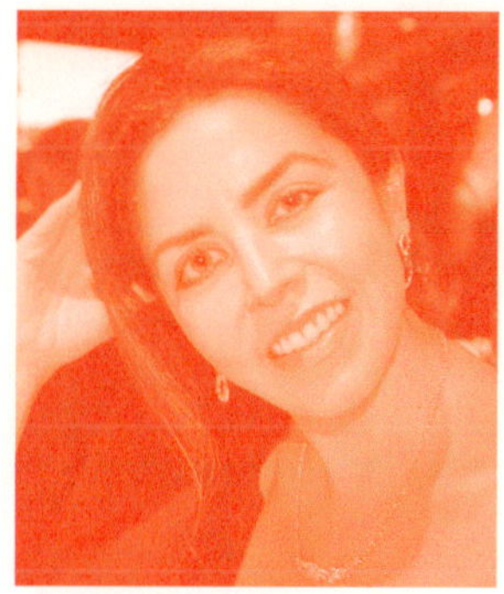

Supporting open minds since 2005

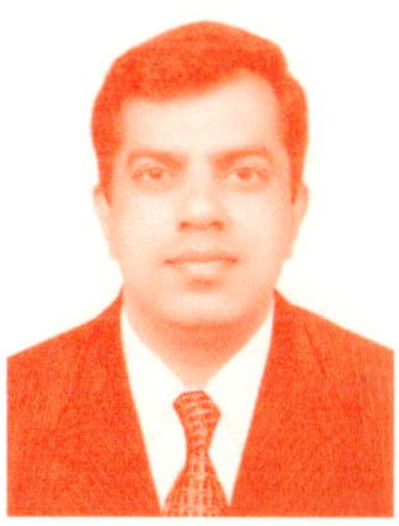
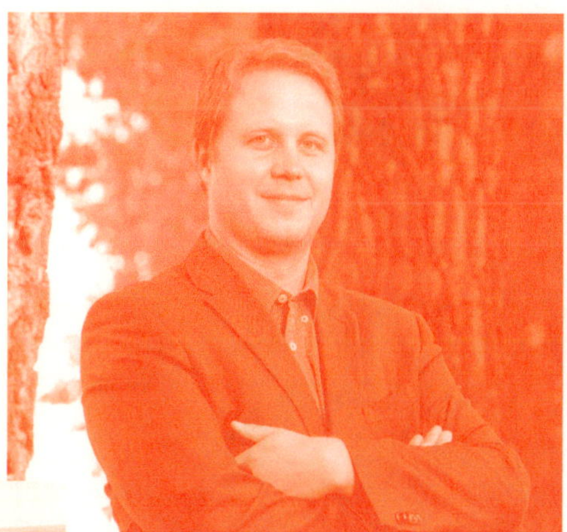
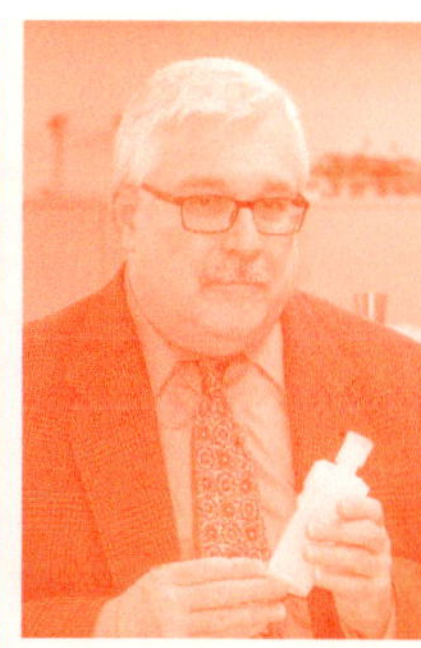
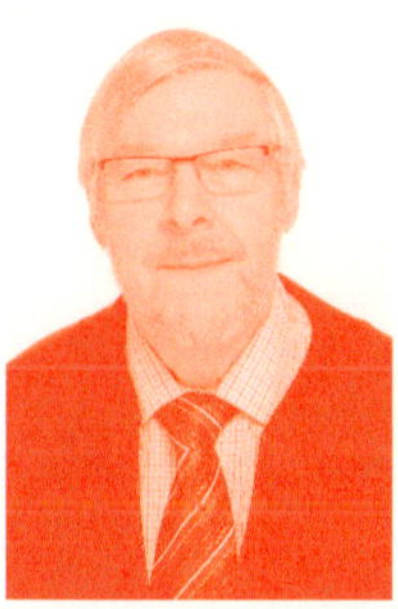
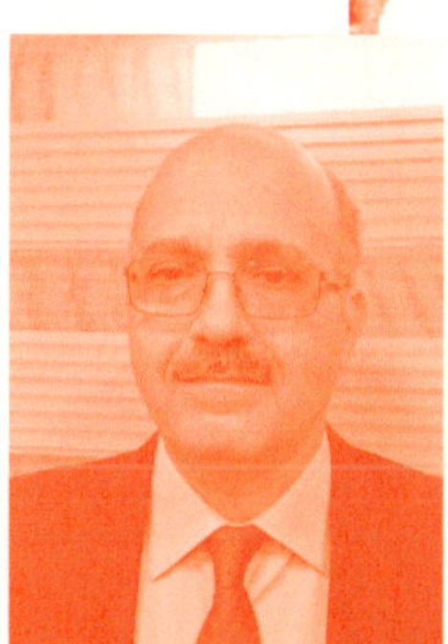
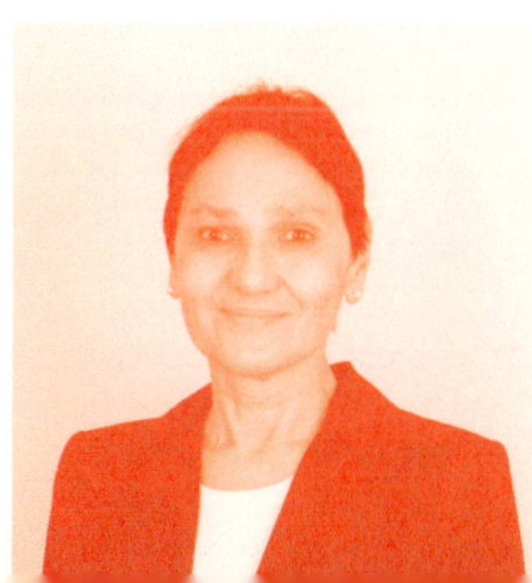
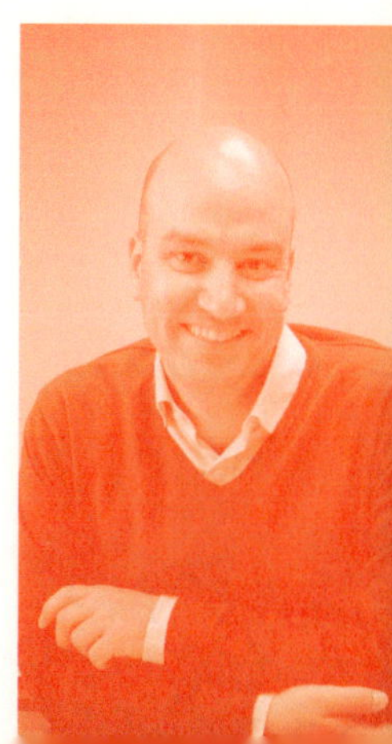

Dysphagia - New Advances
http://dx.doi.org/10.5772/intechopen.95743
Edited by Monjur Ahmed

Contributors
Mary Hägg, Natalie R. Morris, José Luis Braga de Aquino, Vania Aparecida Leandro-Merhi, Prasit Mahawongkajit, Ghazwan Abdulla Hasan, Oscar L. Alves, Isabelle Germain, M.W.M van den Brekel, L. Van Der Molen, Marise Neijman, R.T. Karsten, O. Lapid, Alexandra V. Yakovleva, Alexandr E. Shestopalov, Marina V. Petrova, Pranil Pradhan, Alexey A. Yakovlev, Abdorreza Naser Moghadasi, Fereshteh Ghadiri, Juan Francisco Merino-Torres, Maria Argente-Pla, Katherine Garcia Malpartida, Andrea Micó García, Silvia Martín Sanchis

First published in London, United Kingdom, 2022 by IntechOpen
IntechOpen is the global imprint of INTECHOPEN LIMITED, registered in England and Wales, registration number: 11086078, 5 Princes Gate Court, London, SW7 2QJ, United Kingdom
Printed in Croatia

British Library Cataloguing-in-Publication Data
A catalogue record for this book is available from the British Library

Additional hard and PDF copies can be obtained from orders@intechopen.com

Dysphagia - New Advances
Edited by Monjur Ahmed
p. cm.
Print ISBN 978-1-78985-409-1
Online ISBN 978-1-78985-410-7
eBook (PDF) ISBN 978-1-83962-510-7

For EU product safety concerns:
IN TECH d.o.o., Prolaz Marije Krucifikse Kozulić 3, 51000 Rijeka, Croatia, info@intechopen.com or visit our website at intechopen.com.

Meet the editor

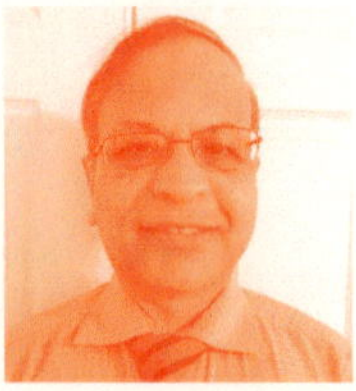

Monjur Ahmed, MD, FRCP, is an Associate Professor of Medicine, at the Thomas Jefferson University, Philadelphia, Pennsylvania, USA. He has been a practicing gastroenterologist for twenty-four years. He has a special interest in biliary diseases, gastrointestinal bleeding, colon cancer, inflammatory bowel disease, eosinophilic esophagitis, gastrointestinal motility disorders, and dysphagia. He also serves as an editor-in-chief of the *World Journal of Gastrointestinal Oncology*.

Contents

Preface

This is a unique book that gives an update on the management of dysphagia due to various disorders. It discusses both the diagnostic and therapeutic aspects of dysphagia. Management of dysphagia due to corrosive ingestion can be challenging. In the chapter on acute management in corrosive ingestion, the author describes the Zargar classification and step-by-step management. Postoperative dysphagia following anterior cervical spinal surgery is common. In the chapter on this topic, the authors review this clinical problem's pathogenesis and provide perioperative and postoperative recommendations. In a chapter on amyotrophic lateral sclerosis, the authors describe the different mechanisms of dysphagia in this disease. Although dysphagia is managed endoscopically or surgically most of the time, nutritional management is also extremely important, particularly in neurogenic and neuromuscular diseases. A chapter on this subject reviews the different nutritional supports in neurogenic dysphagia in detail. Another chapter examines the role of surgery in patients with advanced achalasia and esophageal diameter of 6 cm or more. Patients with head and neck cancer develop dysphagia after radiation and surgical treatment. Lipofilling is a technique of autologous transplantation of fat from one place to another. One chapter describes the role of lipofilling in head and neck cancer patients who develop post-treatment dysphagia. The mechanism of dysphagia in neuroinflammatory diseases of the central nervous system is complex. Another chapter presents the pathophysiology, clinical assessment, and treatment of dysphagia in this category of patients. IQoro is a clinically effective oral neuromuscular treatment for dysphagia due to stroke and cerebral palsy. It activates all the muscles for swallowing. The final chapter describes this treatment in detail. This book is a useful reference for physicians, surgeons, speech therapists, and nutritionists involved in managing dysphagia.

Monjur Ahmed, MD, FRCP
Thomas Jefferson University,
Philadelphia, USA

Section 1

Dysphagia Due to Chemical Injury

Chapter 1

Acute Management in Corrosive Ingestion

Prasit Mahawongkajit

Abstract

Corrosive ingestion is an important health problem and medical emergency worldwide. It occurs by accident or by intention. Acids cause coagulation necrosis, and alkalis cause liquefaction necrosis. In the acute period, stabilization of the patient is most important. Airway assessment and prompt management are a priority for severe cases. Caustic substance reflux into the esophagus resulting in further damage should be prevented. The initial evaluation should be performed by endoscopy and graded according to the Zargar classification. Computed tomography (CT) should be used to assess injury to the esophagus because CT is non-invasive. For Zargar 3b injuries, views from both endoscopy and CT scans should be considered. Post-corrosive esophageal stricture is a complication that responds poorly to treatment. Research and development for stricture prevention are ongoing, especially for Zargar 2b and 3a cases.

Keywords: corrosive esophageal injury, caustic injury, esophageal perforation, post-corrosive esophageal stricture

1. Introduction

Corrosive ingestion is a medical emergency that is especially prevalent in developing countries such as Thailand [1–9]. Since 2020, the COVID-19 has had an enormous impact on many sectors worldwide, and it had affected the trend of rising incidence and severity of diseases [10]. However, the actual incidence should not be precise as the tip of the iceberg phenomenon is probably under-report [4, 8]. Currently, various studies on this topic are still being developed for medical knowledge to the achievement goal of the best practice. Perforation and stricture are complications of corrosive ingestion which are currently being researched and which are discussed in this chapter.

2. Cause of injury

Caustic injuries are caused by the ingestion of substances with acid or base properties. Acids cause coagulation necrosis, and alkalis cause liquefaction necrosis. Corrosive ingestion in children is usually accidental. In adults, it might be related to suicide. Therefore, it is a public health concern with mental and socioeconomic aspects [1, 2, 6, 11].

3. Impact of corrosive injury

Morbidity with mortality rates of corrosive injuries are high [12, 13]. Airway assessment and prompt management are priorities in emergency settings, especially in severe cases [2, 13, 14]. Extensive burns can cause the fragile esophageal wall to become perforated. Physicians must evaluate this condition as soon as possible. Stricture is another complication that physicians need to evaluate. Post-corrosive esophageal strictures cause patients to suffer and are difficult to treat [2–4, 9, 12, 15–19].

4. Pathophysiology

Caustic substances with pH less than two or more than 12 are especially destructive. Form, concentration, amount of ingestion, and contact duration also affect the results. Acidic substances generate coagulation necrosis which creates eschar formation. Eschar can limit the penetration of injuries [16]. On the other hand, alkaline substances melt the tissue protein and initiate liquefactive necrosis with saponification that can penetrate deeper into the esophageal wall [17].

Perforation occurs in the acute stage of severe esophageal injuries. As a consequence of perforation, stricture follows during the recovery stage. Tissue injuries after corrosive ingestion go through three phases. Phase 1 is characterized by cell necrosis and thrombosis, 48–72 hours after the event. Next, in Phase 2, there is mucosal sloughing with ulceration of the esophageal wall plus fibroblast colonization and granulation. This phase continues for 14 days from the Phase 1, and the esophagus is friable during this phase. Finally, in Phase 3, the healing process starts in the third week and usually continues 3–6 months [3, 20, 21].

5. Management

When patients arrive at the emergency department, stabilization of the patient is the most important target for this stage [21]. Signs and symptoms that often occur in corrosive ingested patients include burning of the oral cavity, drooling, nausea, and vomiting. Upper gastrointestinal bleeding can be found in severe cases, indicating substance injuries to the alimentary tract. Respiratory trauma can result in hoarseness, difficulty to breathe, stridor, and airway compromise. Esophagus perforation can be expressed as mediastinitis, chest wall emphysema, and pneumothorax, depending on time and severity.

Physicians should first examine the airway, especially for signs of aspiration or laryngeal injury. Physical examination and history taking should be done for details of the corrosive substance, the volume, timing before admission, pre-hospital treatment, and cause of ingestion. The patient should be given nil per os (NPO) and adequate resuscitation. Nasogastric tube intubation, gastric lavage, administration of emetic drugs, and neutralizing agents are not recommended because reflux of these agents into the esophagus could result in further damage [1, 8, 21]. Intravenous broad-spectrum antibiotics may benefit a patient with high-grade esophageal injuries. The investigation by chest and abdominal radiography should be evaluated. In cases of attempted suicide, the patient should be evaluated by the psychiatric department [1, 3, 4, 9, 22, 23].

The initial evaluation of the severity of a caustic injury provides important information. Esophagogastroduodenoscopy (EGD) is recommended for grading esophageal injuries following the Zargar classification (**Table 1**). Zargar classification can assist prognosis and guide clinical management [16]. The EGD should be done as soon as possible within 24–48 hours. Performing endoscopy after 48 hours

Zargar classification	Description
Grade 0	Normal finding on endoscopic examination
Grade 1	Edema and hyperemia of the mucosa
Grade 2a	Friability, blisters, exudates, hemorrhages, whitish membrane, erosions, and superficial ulceration
Grade 2b	Grade 2a plus deep discrete or circumferential ulceration
Grade 3a	Small scattered areas of multiple ulceration and areas of necrosis with brown-black or grayish discoloration
Grade 3b	Extensive necrosis

Table 1.
Zargar classification of corrosive esophageal injury.

Score	Endoscopic score [16]	Computerized tomography score [24]
0	Grade 0; Normal	Normal
I	Grade 1; Edema and hyperemia of the mucosa	No definite swelling of esophagus wall (<3 mm, within normal limit)
II	Grade 2a; Friability, blisters, exudates, hemorrhages, whitish membrane, erosion, and superficial ulceration	Edematous wall thickening (>3 mm) without periesophageal soft tissue infiltration
	Grade 2b; Grade 2a plus deep discrete or circumferential ulceration	
III	Grade 3a; Small scattered areas of multiple ulceration and areas of necrosis with brown-black or grayish discoloration	Edematous wall thickening with periesophageal soft tissue infiltration pulse well-demarcated tissue interface
	Grade 3b; Extensive necrosis	
VI	Grade 4; Perforation	Edematous wall thickening with periesophageal soft tissue infiltration plus blurring of tissue interface or localized fluid collection around the esophagus or the descending aorta

Table 2.
Endoscopic score and computerized tomography score of corrosive esophageal injury.

is not recommended because the tissue injuries go through Phase 2 when they should not be subjected to an unwanted event [16, 21]. For patients with Zargar grade 1 and 2a, an oral diet may be given. Patients with Zargar grade 2b and 3a can start an oral diet once they can swallow saliva. Esophagectomy should be performed on patients with Zargar grade 3b injuries.

The method for assessing the degree of esophageal damage by computed tomography (CT) with scoring was recently established as a noninvasive modality [24]. Nowadays, the use of CT scans of the chest and abdomen is increasing. CT can assist prognosis after ingestion, but it is still inconclusive [25–27]. CT also provides extraesophageal information regarding anatomies such as the mediastinum, lung, and pleural cavity, which endoscopies do not (**Table 2**).

6. Perforation

Although an endoscopy is an important tool for initial evaluation, contraindications are suspected perforation, oral cavity necrosis, and airway injury with compromised respiration. CT scans can safely provide details about esophageal transmural necrosis consisting of esophageal wall blurring, peri-esophageal fat stranding, and no enhancement of esophageal wall after administration of intravenous contrast [24]. Recent studies reported that unnecessary esophagectomy following endoscopic evaluation of patients with Zargar grade 3b could have been avoided if CT had been used [28–30].

Both CT and endoscopy have distinctive advantages. CT is minimally invasive with high sensitivity and specificity [24, 25, 27–30]. Intra-luminal evaluation by endoscopy reveals subtle details of the esophageal mucosa and degrees of damage [31]. The combination of CT and endoscopy is especially useful for examining patients with Zargar 3b injuries [8, 30, 31].

7. Stricture

As the esophagus is healing following ingestion of a corrosive substance, the possibility of stricture should be assessed. Post-corrosive esophageal stricture is a complication that produces suffering for victims [9, 15, 17]. Esophageal dilation is a therapeutic intervention of choice to perform at the onset of stricture. If left until later, the procedure becomes more difficult, decreasing the success and increasing adverse events [21, 32–36]. Esophageal dilatation can be performed repeatedly according to schedule and using various dilators such as Maloney-Hurst, Savary-Gilliard, and Balloon dilator under the endoscopy, fluoroscopy, or both. Alternative

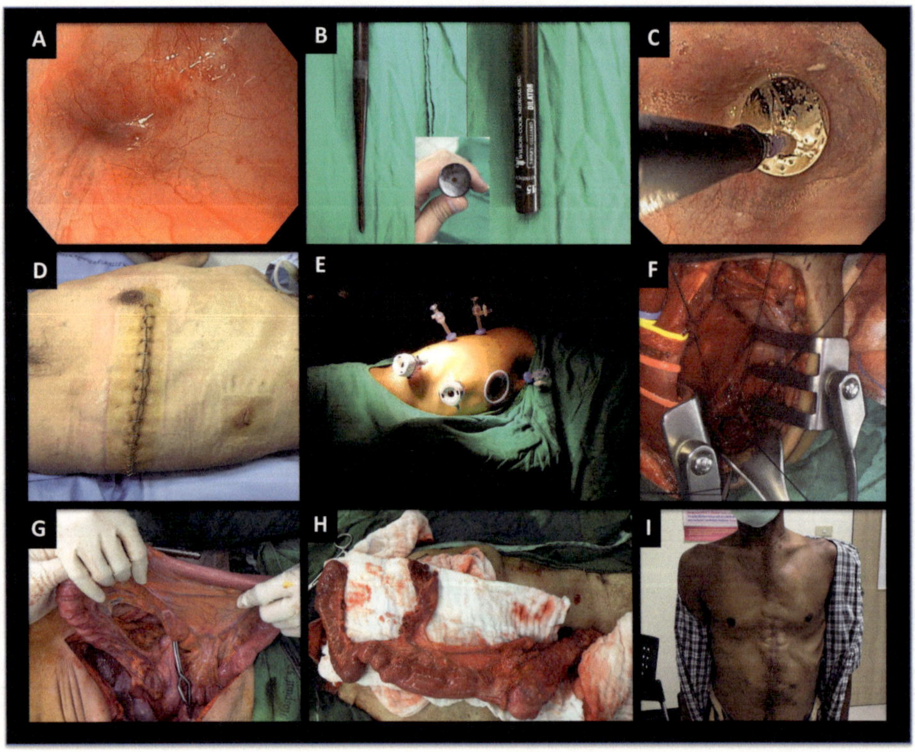

Figure 1.
The treatment options for post-corrosive esophageal stricture. (A) Severe post-corrosive esophageal stricture; (B) Savary-Gilliard dilator; (C) endoscopic balloon dilation; (D) esophagectomy with open right thoracotomy; (E) esophagectomy with video-assisted thoracoscopic surgery (VATS); (F) reconstruction with cervical anastomosis after esophagectomy; (G, H) right side colonic conduit for esophageal replacement; and (I) subcutaneous colon interposition.

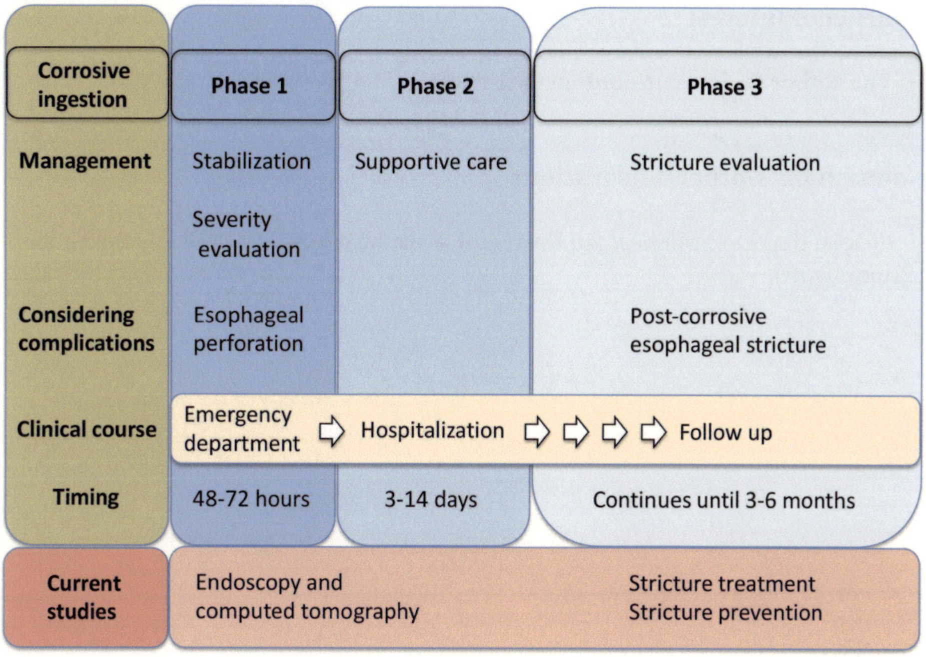

Figure 2.
Schematic diagram of corrosive ingestion in esophageal injury.

methods for post-corrosive esophageal stricture such as esophageal stenting [21, 37, 38], intralesional steroids [21, 39–43], and, Mitomycin-C [21, 44–48] have been published with various outcomes. These options might supplement dilation with better results. In cases of severe stricture, failure to dilate, or refractory strictures, surgery might be necessary (**Figure 1**) [4, 18, 19, 49–54].

Post-corrosive esophageal stricture should highly consider inpatient with Zargar grade 2b and 3a [4, 5, 8, 9, 16, 55]. Although various treatment strategies have been developed, none of them can provide outstanding results. Stricture prevention would be the ideal method. Corticosteroids reduce inflammation, but the benefit is inconclusive. Steroids cause severe adverse side effects such as esophageal candidiasis, gastric ulcer, ethmoiditis, ostcomyelitis, and osteoporosis [56–58]. Recent studies have demonstrated that omeprazole with proton pump inhibitor activity could enhance healing, reduce stricture, and reduce the short-term risk of developing esophageal stricture in patients with 2b and 3a corrosive injuries [9, 59–61]. However, further studies of omeprazole are needed to corroborate these findings (**Figure 2**).

8. Conclusion

Corrosive ingestion is a serious medical emergency that is a global problem, especially in several developing countries. When patients arrive at the emergency department, stabilization of the patient is initially the most important target. Airway assessment and prompt management are the priorities for emergency settings, especially in severe cases. Any intervention that might cause substance reflux into the esophagus resulting in further damage is not recommended. Current methods for assessing the degree of esophageal damage are early endoscopy for Zargar classification and CT scan, which focuses on ruling out perforation. Post-corrosive esophageal stricture can be a consequent complication with poor treatment outcomes, and stricture prevention is an interesting idea.

Conflict of interest

The author declares no conflict of interest.

Notes/thanks/other declarations

Special thanks to Michael Jan Everts for assistance in editing the English version of this chapter.

Author details

Prasit Mahawongkajit
Department of Surgery, Faculty of Medicine, Thammasat University, Pathumthani, Thailand

*Address all correspondence to: prasit_md@yahoo.com

References

[1] Chirica M, Kelly MD, Siboni S, et al. Esophageal emergencies: WSES guidelines. World Journal of Emergency Surgery: WJES. 2019;**14**:26. DOI: 10.1186/s13017-019-0245-2

[2] Hoffman RS, Burns MM, Gosselin S. Ingestion of caustic substances. The New England Journal of Medicine. 2020;**382**(18):1739-1748. DOI: 10.1056/NEJMra1810769

[3] Kalayarasan R, Ananthakrishnan N, Kate V. Corrosive ingestion. Indian Journal of Critical Care Medicine. 2019;**23**(Suppl 4):S282-S286. DOI: 10.5005/jp-journals-10071-23305

[4] Contini S, Scarpignato C. Caustic injury of the upper gastrointestinal tract: A comprehensive review. World Journal of Gastroenterology. 2013;**19**(25):3918-3930. DOI: 10.3748/wjg.v19.i25.3918

[5] Havanond C. Is there a difference between the management of grade 2b and 3 corrosive gastric injuries? Journal of the Medical Association of Thailand. 2002;**85**(3):340-344

[6] Havanond C. Clinical features of corrosive ingestion. Journal of the Medical Association of Thailand. 2003;**86**(10):918-924

[7] Havanond C, Havanond P. Initial signs and symptoms as prognostic indicators of severe gastrointestinal tract injury due to corrosive ingestion. The Journal of Emergency Medicine. 2007;**33**(4):349-353. DOI: 10.1016/j.jemermed.2007.02.062

[8] Chirica M, Bonavina L, Kelly MD, Sarfati E, Cattan P. Caustic ingestion. Lancet. 2017;**389**(10083):2041-2052. DOI: 10.1016/S0140-6736(16)30313-0

[9] Mahawongkajit P, Tomtitchong P, Boochangkool N, et al. Risk factors for esophageal stricture in grade 2b and 3a corrosive esophageal injuries. Journal of Gastrointestinal Surgery. 2018;**22**(10):1659-1664. DOI: 10.1007/s11605-018-3822-x

[10] Thongchuam C, Mahawongkajit P, Kanlerd A. The effect of the COVID-19 on corrosive ingestion in Thailand. Open Access Emergency Medicine. 2021;**13**:299-304. DOI: 10.2147/OAEM.S321218

[11] Li Y, Langworthy J, Xu L, Cai H, Yang Y, Lu Y, et al. Nationwide estimate of emergency department visits in the United States related to caustic ingestion. Diseases of the Esophagus. 2020;**33**(6):doaa012. DOI: 10.1093/dote/doaa012

[12] Alipour Faz A, Arsan F, Peyvandi H, et al. Epidemiologic features and outcomes of caustic ingestions: A 10-year cross-sectional study. Emergency (Tehran, Iran). 2017;**5**(1):e56

[13] Struck MF, Beilicke A, Hoffmeister A, et al. Acute emergency care and airway management of caustic ingestion in adults: Single center observational study. Scandinavian Journal of Trauma, Resuscitation and Emergency Medicine. 2016;**24**:45. DOI: 10.1186/s13049-016-0240-5

[14] Bird JH, Kumar S, Paul C, Ramsden JD. Controversies in the management of caustic ingestion injury: An evidence-based review. Clinical Otolaryngology. 2017;**42**(3):701-708. DOI: 10.1111/coa.12819

[15] Zargar SA, Kochhar R, Nagi B, Mehta S, Mehta SK. Ingestion of corrosive acids. Spectrum of injury to upper gastrointestinal tract and natural history. Gastroenterology. 1989;**97**(3):702-707

[16] Zargar SA, Kochhar R, Mehta S, Mehta SK. The role of fiberoptic endoscopy in the management of corrosive ingestion and modified endoscopic classification of burns. Gastrointestinal Endoscopy. 1991;**37**(2):165-169. DOI: 10.1016/s0016-5107(91)70678-0

[17] Zargar SA, Kochhar R, Nagi B, Mehta S, Mehta SK. Ingestion of strong corrosive alkalis: Spectrum of injury to upper gastrointestinal tract and natural history. The American Journal of Gastroenterology. 1992;**87**(3):337-341

[18] Awsakulsutthi S, Havanond C. A retrospective study of anastomotic leakage between patients with and without vascular enhancement of esophageal reconstructions with colon interposition: Thammasat University Hospital experience. Asian Journal of Surgery. 2015;**38**(3):145-149. DOI: 10.1016/j.asjsur.2015.01.005

[19] Mahawongkajit P, Boochangkool N. Comparison of preoperative CT colonography and colonoscopy for esophageal reconstruction with colonic interposition. Surgery Research and Practice. 2020;**2020**:6585762. DOI: 10.1155/2020/6585762

[20] Osman M, Russell J, Shukla D, Moghadamfalahi M, Granger DN. Responses of the murine esophageal microcirculation to acute exposure to alkali, acid, or hypochlorite. Journal of Pediatric Surgery. 2008;**43**(9):1672-1678. DOI: 10.1016/j.jpedsurg.2008.01.069

[21] Methasate A, Lohsiriwat V. Role of endoscopy in caustic injury of the esophagus. World Journal of Gastrointestinal Endoscopy. 2018;**10**(10):274-282. DOI: 10.4253/wjge.v10.i10.274

[22] Salzman M, O'Malley RN. Updates on the evaluation and management of caustic exposures. Emergency Medicine Clinics of North America. 2007;**25**(2):459-476. DOI: 10.1016/j.emc.2007.02.007

[23] Bonavina L, Chirica M, Skrobic O, et al. Foregut caustic injuries: Results of the world society of emergency surgery consensus conference. World Journal of Emergency Surgery : WJES. 2015;**10**:44. DOI: 10.1186/s13017-015-0039-0

[24] Ryu HH, Jeung KW, Lee BK, et al. Caustic injury: Can CT grading system enable prediction of esophageal stricture? Clinical Toxicology (Philadelphia, Pa.). 2010;**48**(2):137-142. DOI: 10.3109/15563650903585929

[25] Agarwal A, Srivastava DN, Madhusudhan KS. Corrosive injury of the upper gastrointestinal tract: The evolving role of a radiologist. The British Journal of Radiology. 2020;**93**(1114):20200528. DOI: 10.1259/bjr.20200528

[26] Gupta P, Gulati A, Reddy YR, Samanta J, Kochhar R. Does esophageal wall thickness on computed tomography predict response to endoscopic dilatation in patients with corrosive esophageal strictures? JGH Open. 2019;**3**(5):405-408. DOI: 10.1002/jgh3.12176

[27] Bahrami-Motlagh H, Hadizadeh-Neisanghalb M, Peyvandi H. Diagnostic accuracy of computed tomography scan in detection of upper gastrointestinal tract injuries following caustic ingestion. Emergency (Tehran, Iran). 2017;**5**(1):e61

[28] Chirica M, Resche-Rigon M, et al. Computed tomography evaluation of high-grade esophageal necrosis after corrosive ingestion to avoid unnecessary esophagectomy. Surgical Endoscopy. 2015;**29**(6):1452-1461. DOI: 10.1007/s00464-014-3823-0

[29] Isbister GK, Page CB. Early endoscopy or CT in caustic injuries: A

re-evaluation of clinical practice. Clinical Toxicology (Philadelphia, Pa.). 2011;**49**(7):641-642. DOI: 10.3109/15563650.2011.604035

[30] Chirica M, Resche-Rigon M, Zagdanski AM, et al. Computed tomography evaluation of esophagogastric necrosis after caustic ingestion. Annals of Surgery. 2016;**264**(1):107-113. DOI: 10.1097/SLA.0000000000001459

[31] Bonnici KS, Wood DM, Dargan PI. Should computerised tomography replace endoscopy in the evaluation of symptomatic ingestion of corrosive substances? Clinical Toxicology (Philadelphia, Pa.). 2014;**52**(9):911-925. DOI: 10.3109/15563650.2014.957310

[32] Tharavej C, Pungpapong SU, Chanswangphuvana P. Outcome of dilatation and predictors of failed dilatation in patients with acid-induced corrosive esophageal strictures. Surgical Endoscopy. 2018;**32**(2):900-907. DOI: 10.1007/s00464-017-5764-x

[33] Singhal S, Kar P. Management of acid- and alkali-induced esophageal strictures in 79 adults by endoscopic dilation: 8-years' experience in New Delhi. Dysphagia. 2007;**22**(2):130-134. DOI: 10.1007/s00455-006-9064-1

[34] Ilkin Naharci M, Tuzun A, et al. Effectiveness of bougie dilation for the management of corrosive esophageal strictures. Acta Gastroenterologica Belgica. 2006;**69**(4):372-376

[35] Chiu YC, Liang CM, Tam W, et al. The effects of endoscopic-guided balloon dilations in esophageal and gastric strictures caused by corrosive injuries. BMC Gastroenterology. 2013;**13**:99. DOI: 10.1186/1471-230X-13-99

[36] Kim JH, Song HY, Kim HC, et al. Corrosive esophageal strictures: Long-term effectiveness of balloon dilation in 117 patients. Journal of Vascular and Interventional Radiology. 2008;**19**(5): 736-741. DOI: 10.1016/j.jvir.2008.01.015

[37] Abreu M, Nunes I, Corujeira S, Tavares M, Trindade E, Dias JA. Caustic esophageal stenosis: A case report of endoscopic dilation with a dynamic stent. GE Portuguese Journal of Gastroenterology. 2016;**23**(4):218-223. DOI: 10.1016/j.jpge.2015.12.006

[38] Kochhar R, Samanta J, Basha J, et al. Biodegradable stents for caustic esophageal strictures: Do they work? Dysphagia. 2017;**32**(4):575-582. DOI: 10.1007/s00455-017-9800-8

[39] Kochhar R, Ray JD, Sriram PV, Kumar S, Singh K. Intralesional steroids augment the effects of endoscopic dilation in corrosive esophageal strictures. Gastrointestinal Endoscopy. 1999;**49**(4 Pt 1):509-513. DOI: 10.1016/s0016-5107(99)70052-0

[40] Kochhar R, Makharia GK. Usefulness of intralesional triamcinolone in treatment of benign esophageal strictures. Gastrointestinal Endoscopy. 2002;**56**(6):829-834. DOI: 10.1067/mge.2002.129871

[41] Nijhawan S, Udawat HP, Nagar P. Aggressive bougie dilatation and intralesional steroids is effective in refractory benign esophageal strictures secondary to corrosive ingestion. Diseases of the Esophagus. 2016;**29**(8): 1027-1031. DOI: 10.1111/dote.12438

[42] Szapáry L, Tinusz B, Farkas N, et al. Intralesional steroid is beneficial in benign refractory esophageal strictures: A meta-analysis. World Journal of Gastroenterology. 2018;**24**(21):2311-2319. DOI: 10.3748/wjg.v24.i21.2311

[43] Randhawa FA, Butt NF, Talat SO, Sabir SH, Qamar MA. Effectiveness of intralesional steroid injections with dilatation in corrosive oesophageal strictures—A randomized control trial.

The Journal of the Pakistan Medical Association. 2018;**68**(11):1556-1559

[44] Nagaich N, Nijhawan S, Katiyar P, Sharma R, Rathore M. Mitomycin-C: 'a ray of hope' in refractory corrosive esophageal strictures. Diseases of the Esophagus. 2014;**27**(3):203-205. DOI: 10.1111/dote.12092

[45] Méndez-Nieto CM, Zarate-Mondragón F, Ramírez-Mayans J, Flores-Flores M. Topical mitomycin C versus intralesional triamcinolone in the management of esophageal stricture due to caustic ingestion. Revista de Gastroenterología de México. 2015;**80**(4):248-254. DOI: 10.1016/j.rgmx.2015.07.006

[46] El-Asmar KM, Hassan MA, Abdelkader HM, Hamza AF. Topical mitomycin C can effectively alleviate dysphagia in children with long-segment caustic esophageal strictures. Diseases of the Esophagus. 2015;**28**(5): 422-427. DOI: 10.1111/dote.12218

[47] Ghobrial CM, Eskander AE. Prospective study of the effect of topical application of mitomycin C in refractory pediatric caustic esophageal strictures. Surgical Endoscopy. 2018;**32**(12):4932-4938. DOI: 10.1007/s00464-018-6253-6

[48] Flor MM, Ribeiro IB, DE Moura DTH, Marques SB, Bernardo WM, DE Moura EGH. Efficacy of endoscopic topical mitomycin C application in caustic esophageal strictures in the pediatric population: A systematic review and meta-analysis of randomized controlled trials. Arquivos de Gastroenterologia. 2021;**58**(2):253-261. DOI: 10.1590/S0004-2803.202100000-38

[49] Harlak A, Yigit T, Coskun K, et al. Surgical treatment of caustic esophageal strictures in adults. International Journal of Surgery. 2013;**11**(2):164-168. DOI: 10.1016/j.ijsu.2012.12.010

[50] Okonta KE, Tettey M, Abubakar U. In patients with corrosive oesophageal stricture for surgery, is oesophagectomy rather than bypass necessary to reduce the risk of oesophageal malignancy? Interactive Cardiovascular and Thoracic Surgery. 2012;**15**(4):713-715. DOI: 10.1093/icvts/ivs320

[51] Nayar R, Varshney V, Suman S, Soni S, Kumar N. Thoracolaparoscopic-assisted esophagectomy for corrosive-induced esophageal stricture. Cureus. 2020;**12**(5):e7909. DOI: 10.7759/cureus.7909

[52] Gurram RP, Kalayarasan R, Gnanasekaran S, Pottakkat B. Minimally invasive retrosternal esophageal bypass using a mid-colon esophagocoloplasty for corrosive-induced esophageal stricture. World Journal of Surgery. 2020;**44**(12):4153-4160. DOI: 10.1007/s00268-020-05719-4

[53] Knezević JD, Radovanović NS, Simić AP, et al. Colon interposition in the treatment of esophageal caustic strictures: 40 years of experience. Diseases of the Esophagus. 2007;**20**(6): 530-534. DOI: 10.1111/j.1442-2050.2007.00694.x

[54] Radovanović N, Simić A, Kotarac M, et al. Colon interposition for pharyngoesophageal postcorrosive strictures. Hepato-Gastroenterology. 2009;**56**(89):139-143

[55] Ain QU, Jamil M, Safian HA, et al. Assessing the degree of acute esophageal injury secondary to corrosive intake: Insights from a public sector hospitals of a developing country. Cureus. 2020;**12**(10):e10858. DOI: 10.7759/cureus.10858

[56] Katibe R, Abdelgadir I, McGrogan P, Akobeng AK. Corticosteroids for preventing caustic esophageal strictures: Systematic review and meta-analysis. Journal of Pediatric Gastroenterology

and Nutrition. 2018;**66**(6):898-902. DOI: 10.1097/MPG.0000000000001852

[57] Usta M, Erkan T, Cokugras FC, et al. High doses of methylprednisolone in the management of caustic esophageal burns. Pediatrics. 2014;**133**(6): E1518-E1524. DOI: 10.1542/peds.2013-3331

[58] Pelclová D, Navrátil T. Do corticosteroids prevent oesophageal stricture after corrosive ingestion? Toxicological Reviews. 2005;**24**(2):125-129. DOI: 10.2165/00139709-200524020-00006

[59] Topaloglu B, Bicakci U, Tander B, et al. Biochemical and histopathologic effects of omeprazole and vitamin E in rats with corrosive esophageal burns. Pediatric Surgery International. 2008;**24**(5):555-560. DOI: 10.1007/s00383-008-2126-8

[60] Cakal B, Akbal E, Köklü S, Babalı A, Koçak E, Taş A. Acute therapy with intravenous omeprazole on caustic esophageal injury: A prospective case series. Diseases of the Esophagus. 2013;**26**(1):22-26. DOI: 10.1111/j.1442-2050.2011.01319.x

[61] Mahawongkajit P, Tomtitchong P, Boochangkool N, Mingmalairak C, Awsakulsutthi S, Havanond C. A prospective randomized controlled trial of omeprazole for preventing esophageal stricture in grade 2b and 3a corrosive esophageal injuries. Surgical Endoscopy. 2021;**35**(6):2759-2764. DOI: 10.1007/s00464-020-07707-0

Section 2

Dysphagia Due to Neurological Disorders

Chapter 2

Dysphagia of Neurological Origin – Amyotrophic Lateral Sclerosis

Maria Argente-Pla, Katherine Garcia-Malpartida, Andrea Micó-García, Silvia Martín-Sanchis and Juan Francisco Merino-Torres

Abstract

Amyotrophic lateral sclerosis (ALS) is a progressive neurodegenerative disorder of unknown etiology that affects upper and lower motor neurons resulting in progressive atrophy of skeletal muscles. There are two forms of ALS: spinal motor neuron injury and bulbar paresis. Dysphagia is a highly prevalent severe and invalidating symptom in ALS: almost 80% of ALS patients with bulbar paresis will develop dysphagia. Also, dysphagia is one of the most common and serious complications, with respiratory insufficiency, in patients with ALS as it exposes them to malnutrition, dehydration and aspiration pneumonia. These conditions are reported to be associated with a minor survival in patients with ALS. Screening for dysphagia must be performed in all ALS patients at diagnosis and during the follow-up to approach dysphagia as soon as possible. This chapter includes the latest developments in the assessment and approach of dysphagia in ALS patients.

Keywords: dysphagia, neurodegenerative disorder, amyotrophic lateral sclerosis, malnutrition, swallowing

1. Introduction

Amyotrophic lateral sclerosis (ALS) is a neurodegenerative disease that characteristically affects the upper motor neuron (located in the motor cortex) and the lower motor neuron (located in the brainstem and medullary anterior horn). As a consequence, muscular weakness ensues, which progresses to paralysis, spreading from one body region to another in a way that affects motor autonomy, oral communication, swallowing and breathing [1]. ALS is an irreversible, disabling chronic disease with serious complications.

ALS is the third neurodegenerative disease in incidence, after dementia and Parkinson's disease. It is, together with its variants, primary lateral sclerosis, progressive muscular atrophy, and progressive bulbar palsy, the most common motor neuron disease in adults. The incidence of ALS is between 1.5 and 2.5 new cases per 100,000 inhabitants per year, and the prevalence is between 4 and 6 people per 100,000 inhabitants, being relatively uniform in Western countries [2, 3].

The diagnosis of ALS is currently based on the Awaji criteria [4], respectively, the revised El-Escorial criteria [5]. Also, the Gold-Coast criteria have recently been proposed [6].

ALS occurs in two main forms: the central or bulbar form, also known as progressive bulbar palsy, and the peripheral or spinal form. In bulbar ALS, at least 80% of patients will develop dysarthria and dysphagia [7], while in the spinal or peripheral form, muscle weakness predominates, although dysphagia may appear in the evolutionary course.

Currently, there is no curative treatment, but there are some effective measures to prolong patient survival, such as nutritional management, whose aim is the prevention of malnutrition and the improvement of quality of life. Riluzole is the only medication approved for treatment of ALS by the United States Food and Drug Administration and the European Medicine Agency. Its mechanism of action is complex and includes inhibition of glutamate release, blocking of receptors for excitatory amino acids, inactivation of voltage-gated sodium channels, and stimulation of a G-protein-dependent signal transduction. Riluzole is generally well tolerated and may prolong survival by 2–3 months [8]. Recent reports suggest that riluzole could increase the survival of patients with ALS for up to 19 months [9].

Nonetheless, survival of ALS patients from diagnosis is 20% at five years after diagnosis of the disease [10]: mean survival of ALS is 3–5 years, with 5–10% living longer than 10 years [11]. The main causes of mortality are respiratory failure and malnutrition with dehydration [12, 13].

ALS patients frequently present malnutrition, this being an independent prognostic factor for survival [14]. The causes of malnutrition are the appearance of dysphagia, whose prevalence reaches 80% in the evolutionary course of ALS, as well as the decrease in intake due to loss of autonomy, muscle atrophy, fatigue and increased energy requirements.

The prevalence of malnutrition varies from 16 to 53% depending on the parameters used [15], the form of presentation of the disease and the moment in its evolutionary course. Therefore, a nutritional assessment is recommended in all patients diagnosed with ALS, whether bulbar or spinal, at the time of diagnosis of the disease [12].

The follow-up and nutritional approach of these patients is chronic, without considering the possibility of discharge or end of follow-up. However, there are no precise premises regarding follow-up (frequency of visits) [12]. Furthermore, it is important to bear in mind that the management of these patients is multidisciplinary (Pneumology, Neurology, Rehabilitation, etc.) and requires closer surveillance than other types of patients.

Swallowing is a complex act that relies on the correct coordination of motor and sensory systems of oral, pharyngeal and esophageal strictures. Dysphagia is defined as the difficulty in passing the food bolus from the mouth to the stomach caused by the anatomical or functional alteration of various structures involved in swallowing. It includes the behavioral, sensory and motor alterations that occur during swallowing, including the state of consciousness prior to the act of eating, the visual recognition of food and the physiological responses to the smell and presence of food.

Swallowing disorders can appear acutely or insidiously and progressively. Dysphagia is classified according to its etiology (mechanical or motor) or according to its location (oropharyngeal or esophageal).

In ALS patients, dysphagia is progressive, motor, and occurs both at the oropharyngeal and esophageal levels. Its prevalence is 30% at diagnosis, with an increasing incidence as the disease evolves, appearing in up to 80% of patients with ALS [7, 12].

The importance in the diagnosis of dysphagia lies in its complications, derived from a decrease in a reduction in the efficacy and safety of swallowing. Complications from dysphagia include malnutrition, dehydration, aspiration and pneumonia. Malnutrition and aspiration increase the risk of death by 7.7 times in ALS patients, hence the importance of its diagnosis and approach [11].

2. Physiopathology of dysphagia: focusing on ALS

Swallowing is a complex act that involves the coordination of multiple sensory and motor systems. During the oral phase, the tongue forms and holds a bolus on the anterior tongue. Currently, the posterior tongue prevents the food from entering the pharynx prematurely. After bolus formation, the posterior transport of the bolus is initiated by the anterior tongue pressing against the hard palate. In the pharyngeal phase, the posterior tongue retracts against the pharyngeal wall and contributes to the downward propulsion of the bolus [16].

ALS may present with a combination of spastic and flaccid weakness that can affect swallowing significantly. Dysphagia in ALS results from bulbar sensory-motor neurodegeneration, which is a pathognomonic feature of ALS [1]. Involvement of the motor nuclei located in the brainstem causes the characteristic bulbar muscle weakness and atrophy, leading to dysphagia. Oropharyngeal impairment of the tongue has been identified, but the underlying mechanisms of its motor dysfunction are not completely understood [17].

Impairment of the tongue seems to represent a major risk factor for aspiration [18]. One study showed a correlation between tongue pressure and the severity of dysphagia and physical performance in 39 patients with ALS [19]. Although swallowing pressures are known to be considerably weaker than maximum pressure exerted by tongue-palate contact pressure tasks, specific measures of maximum tongue strength have been shown to be associated with overall swallowing performance [20].

The occurrence of dysphagia in ALS patients is also related to impairments in the upper aerodigestive tract and respiratory and laryngeal muscles to the extent that they affect the expiratory phase of voluntary cough. There is a strong connection between poor effective voluntary cough and the presence of penetration/aspiration events [21].

One study looked into the pathophysiological mechanisms of dysphagia in 43 patients with sporadic ALS, using clinical and electrophysiological methods that objectively measured the oropharyngeal phase of voluntarily initiated swallowing, and compared them with those obtained from 50 age-matched control subjects [22]. Laryngeal movements were detected by a piezoelectric sensor and muscle electromyography (EMG) of submental muscles, while needle EMG recorded the activity of the cricopharyngeal muscle of the upper esophageal sphincter (UES) during swallowing. ALS patients with dysphagia displayed the following abnormal findings: 1) submental muscle activity of the laryngeal elevators, which produce reflex upward deflection of the larynx during wet swallowing, was significantly prolonged, whereas the laryngeal relocation time of the swallowing reflex remained within normal limits; 2) concerning the cricopharyngeal sphincter muscle, EMG demonstrated severe abnormalities during voluntarily initiated swallows. The opening of the sphincter was delayed and/or the closure occurred prematurely, the total duration of opening was shortened, and, at times, unexpected motor unit bursts appeared during this period; and 3) during voluntarily initiated swallow, there was a significant lack of coordination between the laryngeal elevator muscles and the cricopharyngeal sphincter muscle. These results point at two pathophysiological mechanisms that cause dysphagia in ALS patients: 1) the triggering of the swallowing reflex for the voluntarily initiated swallow is delayed and eventually abolished, whereas the spontaneous reflexive swallows are preserved until the preterminal stage of ALS; 2) the cricopharyngeal sphincter muscle of the UES becomes hyperreflexic and hypertonic. As a result, the laryngeal protective system and the bolus transport system of deglutition lose their coordination during voluntarily initiated swallowing.

Another study investigated the variations of esophageal peristalsis in 28 ALS patients with predominantly bulbar or predominantly pseudobulbar clinical presentation by using esophageal manometry (EM) [23]. Swallowing was initiated with 5–10 mL of water (wet swallows) and saliva (dry swallows) and repeated at 30-second intervals. The manometric parameters were measured automatically and visualized by the computer system. In patients with pseudobulbar presentation, an increase of the resting pressure value in the UES >45 mmHg, a wave-like course of resting pressure, and toothed peristaltic waves were observed. In patients with bulbar presentation, a low amplitude of peristaltic waves <30 mmHg (mean: 17 ± 5) was recorded, without signs of esophageal motility disturbance at onset or during progression. EM procedure allows objectively distinguishing dysphagia in ALS patients due to bulbar syndrome from dysphagia due to pseudobulbar syndrome. It is crucial to identify patients with pseudobulbar clinical presentation due to their high risk of aspiration.

When considering management and treatment of dysphagia, visualization of physiology is the only reliable method to understand the pathophysiology of this condition [24].

3. Dysphagia assessment

The diagnosis of dysphagia is of utmost importance, given the burden of this symptom, causing malnutrition, dehydration, aspiration pneumonia, respiratory failure, and reduced quality of life. Aspiration and malnutrition increase the risk of death [25]. Early identification of dysphagia facilitates improved management, reduced risk of malnutrition and postponed percutaneous endoscopic gastrostomy (PEG) tube placement [26, 27]. The search for dysphagia as early as possible is key in order to prevent its complications.

The diagnosis of dysphagia is more easily performed at multidisciplinary clinics. A dysphagia assessment should be performed in all patients with ALS, both at diagnosis and during follow-up, with a recommended frequency of every 3 months, as part of a complete clinical and neurological evaluation [12].

Dysphagia can be underestimated in ALS due to progressive adaptation to the slow bulbar deterioration and given the inconsistencies in what patients report about the condition. Often, oral stage deficits like difficulties in chewing or oral residue are not reported by the patient until pharyngeal stage deficits, such as coughing or choking, are observed.

A clinical swallow evaluation for suspected dysphagia involves medical history, physical inspection of swallowing, instrumental evaluation, pulmonary function, and bulbar function. However, most importantly, a screening test for dysphagia should be carried out.

Medical history. This includes the reporting of symptoms related to dysphagia, kind of diet, assistance with feeding, changes in body weight, coughing or choking with meals, length of time needed for food intake and saliva management. A validated questionnaire to assess these symptoms is the Eating assessment tool 10 (EAT-10), which has been validated for use in ALS [27]. This study reported high clinical utility and ability to detect aspiration risk in ALS (86% sensitivity, 76% specificity and 95% negative predictive value). However, the validation of the test was performed only against penetration and aspiration scores on the videofluoroscopic swallowing study (VFSS) and not against any overall parameter of swallowing efficiency and safety. The kind of diet can be evaluated by the Neuromuscular Disease Swallowing Status Scale (NdSSS) and the Swallowing subscale on Amyotrophic Lateral Sclerosis Severity Scale (ALSSS). However, these scales do not detect all the patients with alterations in swallowing [28]. An important parameter related to dysphagia and intake is weight loss, which is, therefore, mandatorily recorded at all visits. Moreover, it is important to remember that weight loss and dietary intake are associated with more than just dysphagia.

Physical inspection of systems involved in swallowing and swallowing musculature should go beyond the mere observation of swallowing competence with test swallows. A dysphagia/aspiration screening evaluation is useful when determining the dysphagia risk; however, only limited validation has been completed in ALS. One study validated the volume-viscosity swallowing test (V-VST) against VFSS in 20 ALS patients and reported 93% sensitivity and 80% specificity, respectively [29]. The V-VST is a screening evaluation that involves determining safety and efficiency of swallowing, following the administration of multiple volumes and viscosities of liquids. Another method is the sequential water swallowing (SWS), which involves drinking 100 ml of water in a single, uninterrupted swallow. One study reported that 43% of patients with ALS have a disorganized pattern in their sequential swallows [30].

Instrumental evaluation, such as VFSS or functional endoscopic evaluation of swallow (FEES), is used to visualize the swallowing physiology. These techniques are essential and are the most commonly used, being considered the gold standard in the exploration of dysphagia in ALS, due to the high risk for silent aspiration that these patients have. In fact, one study suggests that up to 55% of ALS patients may present with silent aspiration [31]. VFSS can be used to evaluate problems in the oral phase of the swallowing process, and intradeglutitive silent aspiration can be detected. The interpretation of VFSS results can be done with the videofluoroscopic dysphagia scale (VDS), which contains 14 categories that represent oral functions (lip closure, mastication, bolus formation, premature bolus loss, apraxia, and oral transit time) and pharyngeal functions (pharyngeal triggering, laryngeal elevation, epiglottic closure, pharyngeal transit time, pharyngeal coating, vallecular and pyriform sinus residues, and tracheal aspiration) [32]. A modified version of VSD (mVSD) has been developed to overcome low inter-rater reliability of some categories in the VDS [33]. FEES is a valid, repeatable, and low-cost alternative, used to directly visualize the swallowing process and the saliva movement, and it is able to evaluate pharyngo-laryngeal sensitivity in addition to motility [34]. Other instrumental methods are manometry, in addition to VFSS, electromyography of submental, laryngeal, pharyngeal and diaphragmatic nerves, esophageal scintography [35], tongue sonography and electromagnetic articulography.

Pulmonary function, generally assessed with forced vital capacity (FVC) and cough function, must be explored in patients with dysphagia. Patients with deteriorated pulmonary function are more likely to aspirate.

Bulbar function consists of the evaluation of the anatomy and physiology of head and neck structures involved in swallowing, including an evaluation of the cranial nerves essential for swallowing. The Centre for Neurologic Study Bulbar Function Scale (CNS-BFS) is a useful metric for assessing bulbar function. Among bulbar muscles, the tongue musculature appears to be disproportionally more affected by ALS [36], and tongue strength is a prognostic indicator of survival at the time of ALS diagnosis [37]. Besides, measuring the maximum tongue strength is useful for early detection of dysphagia in ALS [38]. Other important signs of bulbar impairment are weak cough and dysarthria, which should be investigated.

It is imperative to derivate to a speech-language pathologist (SLP) if any bulbar dysfunction is identified. SLP plays an important role in the care of patients with speech, language, or swallowing difficulties that can result from a variety of medical condition.

One of the ways to improve reliability of clinical evaluations is to use standardized and validated protocols. A comprehensive assessment protocol, such as the Mann Assessment of Swallowing Ability (MASA), may be useful to carry out research in the ALS population. MASA, developed and validated for stroke, includes a detailed oral mechanism examination, cranial nerve testing and swallowing function evaluation [39].

Despite this, there is a lack of studies related to the diagnosis of dysphagia in patients with ALS, which is reflected in a significant variability and inconsistency in the management of dysphagia in ALS, as shown in a survey of current clinical practice patterns at 38 ALS centers in the United States in 2017 [40]. In another survey study performed in 2020, 88.9% of SLP performed an instrumental dysphagia evaluation in ALS patients, although the timing of when the evaluation occurred varied significantly; 42.2% of the clinicians carried it out at baseline even prior to the appearance of any bulbar symptoms [41].

4. Dysphagia and nutritional management

4.1 Dysphagia treatment

The aim of dysphagia treatment is to attain an oral diet with safe (to avoid respiratory infections and aspiration pneumonia) and effective swallowing (to maintain an adequate level of nutrition and hydration). Several postural, hygienic and dietary measures must be adopted to achieve this aim along with rehabilitative treatment.

4.1.1 General recommendations

The following postural and hygienic measures are included [42]:

- The environment must be comfortable and calm, which favors concentration, avoiding distractions during the meal.
- Do not start feeding if the patient is sleepy or restless, or if he/she is tired (avoid physical therapy and previous examinations).
- Sufficient time for food intake must be guaranteed.
- The proper position when eating is sitting with one's back straight, feet flat on the floor and the head slightly tilted forward when swallowing. If a person is unable to get out of bed, he/she should be positioned as upright as possible. Food intake should not take place while the head is tilted back.
- Self-feeding is preferable: the patient should feed him–/herself. This reduces the risk of aspiration, but the patient should always be under the supervision of a family member.

- The type of spoon indicated must be used: soup spoon, dessert spoon – candy – or coffee spoon.

- It should be checked that the previous spoonful has been swallowed before another one is given.

- Syringes or straws should not be used.

- Good oral hygiene must be kept to avoid respiratory infections in case of infection. If dentures are worn, they must be in place and tight.

4.1.2 Rehabilitation treatment

Rehabilitation treatment should be carried out whenever possible so that the patient can maintain an adequate oral intake to a greater or lesser extent. Postural maneuvers should be recommended to protect the airway during swallowing [12]. There is no strong evidence in the literature for dysphagia intervention in patients with ALS. Thus, rehabilitation treatment should be individualized. Aspects that influence the selection of the most suitable technique for each patient should be evaluated, such as the patient's cognitive status, behavioral and emotional aspects, degree of fatigue and family support. Based on these criteria, the most rehabilitative technique will be selected for each patient. Some rehabilitation techniques are postural strategies, sensory enhancement strategies (such as mechanical tongue stimulation, bolus changes in volume, temperature, and flavor, thermal stimulation, and changes in taste or acid flavor), neuromuscular practice, compensatory swallowing maneuvers and facilitation techniques.

Some compensatory swallowing maneuvers have been studied in patients with ALS. The chin-tuck posture was found to be useful in most cases, given that it offers a valuable protection mechanism for the airways by opening the valleculae and preventing penetration into the larynx [43]. The indication of the other maneuvers differs according to the mechanism involved in relation to disease characteristics and progression. Thus, hyperextended head posture is indicated in the absence of tongue pumping. If there is hypertonicity, incomplete release, or premature closure of the UES, head rotation is indicated [43]. However, current clinical guidelines do not suggest specific postural maneuvers [12].

Also, saliva could interfere with the management of dysphagia. However, the current evidence to recommend pharmacological treatments such as antimuscarinics in affected patients is low. There is no evidence linking the treatment of saliva issues with the improvement of dysphagia [12].

4.2 Nutritional management

The aim of nutritional management in patients with ALS is to prevent and/or treat malnutrition, to reduce the risk of aspiration, to prevent morbidity and mortality associated with malnutrition and dysphagia, and to improve quality of life. The nutritional approach in these patients includes the early detection of inefficient food intake, the need to adjust the consistency of the diet and, if oral feeding is not possible, the early indication of enteral nutrition by gastrostomy [12].

The nutritional approach modality is carried out according to the clinical situation, being conditioned in these patients by the safety and efficacy of swallowing and by the presence or absence of malnutrition.

In a malnourished patient or a patient being at nutritional risk, in whom oral feeding is possible, the first step is to optimize the diet and reduce the risk of aspiration [12].

The diet must be complete and cover the caloric-protein requirements of each patient. Energy requirements should be estimated as approx. 25–30 and 30 kcal/kg/day in ventilated and non-ventilated ALS patients, respectively [12]. Protein requirements should be calculated at a rate of 1–1.2 g/kg/day [44].

The diet composition for ALS patients does not differ from that of the general population with regard to the recommended macro- and micronutrients distribution [45–50]:

- Proteins: 15–18% of total energy intake.
- Carbohydrates: 55–60% of total energy intake.
- Fats: 30–35% of total energy intake.
- Fiber: fiber-rich diet is recommended, with contributions equal to or greater than 25 g/day.
- Water: it is advisable to ensure a water intake of at least 1 ml/Kcal/day, to prevent dehydration.
- Micronutrients: following the recommendations for the general population according to age and sex of the patient [46–50].

Dietary counseling and modification of food texture is a fundamental aspect of dysphagia treatment. Dietary modification alters the texture of both liquid and solid foods. These modifications should be based on each patient's swallowing capacity and must be regularly evaluated. Dietary modification allows achieving a better nutritional status and better quality of life in patients with special nutritional requirements.

There are multiple recommended methods for modifying the texture of solids and liquids. The *International Dysphagia Diet Standardization Initiative* (IDDSI) [51] establishes five levels of drink thickness (thin plus four levels of thickness) and five levels of food texture (regular plus four levels of modification):

- Texture levels for solid foods: regular, soft, and bite-sized, minced, and moist, pureed and liquidized.
- Texture levels for liquids in the treatment of dysphagia: thin, slightly thick, mildly thick, moderately thick and extremely thick.

Once the diagnosis of dysphagia has been made, the most appropriate solid and liquid food texture for the patient will be established, as well as the volume in which it should be administered.

Dietary modification includes high nutritional value ground or easy-to-swallow diets; texture modifiers, such as thickeners, gel waters or thickened beverages; and diet enhancers (food or nutrient modules) [52]. Also, certain foods should be avoided since they pose a high risk of choking, i.e., foods with double textures, dry or crunchy foods, sticky foods, foods that lose liquid when being chewed, and fibrous and/or filamentary foods.

Thickener modules are products with the ability to thicken, composed of modified starches or gums or a mixture of both, available as powder and with a neutral flavor. They are exclusively intended to increase the consistency of liquid foods. Thickeners composed exclusively of gums preserve the natural appearance of the liquid (unlike those that contain starches) and, therefore, improve the compliance of the patient with dysphagia.

If these dietary modifications do not allow maintaining an adequate nutritional state, oral nutritional supplements (ONS) will be administered, in addition to a modified diet.

Nutritional supplementation is recommended for ALS patients who do not cover their nutritional requirements with an enriched diet. However, there is insufficient data to affirm that oral nutritional supplementation can improve survival in ALS patients [12]. There are no specific formulas for patients with ALS. Hypercaloric formulas with fiber and high viscosity are generally recommended to prevent constipation and reduce the use of thickeners. Thickened ONS have been marketed in recent years and are suitable for patients with difficulties in swallowing, requiring a level 3 consistency or more.

All these measures, together with the general recommendations and the rehabilitative treatment of dysphagia, are aimed at optimizing safe oral intake. However, dysphagia in ALS patients is generally progressive. Thus, if dysphagia makes oral nutritional intake impossible or the patient is severely malnourished, enteral nutrition may be required. Enteral nutrition will preferably be administered by gastrostomy tube [12].

PEG is the most widely technique and is performed under endoscopic control. Its placement and use are well tolerated by the patient and allows them to meet their nutritional needs.

The timing of PEG placement is controversial.

However, there are studies that recommend the placement of a PEG in ALS patients when forced vital capacity is still greater than 50% [53], since a lower percentage would indicate a greater deterioration in lung function that could increase the risk of complications during the procedure. The American Academy of Neurology [54] recommends rejecting gastrostomy when the FVC is below 30% and considers other forms of palliative care. However, several studies show that gastrostomy could be performed safely in patients with insufficient respiratory function [55–57]. The current clinical guidelines [12] do not take a clear position and allow recommendation, respectively, rejection of gastrostomy based on FVC. The reason is that ALS patients with dysphagia, particularly those with primary bulbar involvement, may have poor spirometry performance due to orofacial muscle weakness.

However, early gastrostomy implantation prevents the development of disease complications and improves the quality of life of these patients [58] but has not clearly shown a benefit in patient survival [59]. However, patients who still maintain oral intake tend to be reluctant to place it early.

In any case, the timing of the PEG placement must be agreed with the patient and family, respecting their wishes [12].

5. Conclusions and recommendations

- ALS is a complex disease, and its management requires a multidisciplinary approach that includes the figure of endocrinologists, speech therapists, pharmacists, nurses, nutritionists, and speech therapists.

- The prevalence of malnutrition in patients with ALS is high, in part, due to the high prevalence of dysphagia in these patients.

- A nutritional assessment should be carried out at the diagnosis of the disease and periodically to prevent and treat malnutrition.

- Screening for dysphagia should be performed at the diagnosis of the disease and regularly every 3 months to avoid possible complications.
- Video swallowing is the test of choice for the diagnosis of dysphagia in patients with ALS since it allows early signs to be detected, although V-MECV is a safe and effective alternative.
- The diet must be adapted at all times. The use of dietary counseling and the use of thickeners enables an individualized and safe nutritional intervention, adapting the texture of liquids and solids according to the efficacy and safety of swallowing for each patient.
- ONS can be used to supplement and reinforce the oral diet, making them a useful tool to prevent and treat malnutrition in patients with ALS. However, current legislation does not provide for funding for oral enteral nutrition formulas unless they are administered by tube or ostomy.
- Gastrostomy is a safe method of eating. The time of placement must be agreed with the patient since it is not without risks. There is no specific formula for patients with ALS, but it is recommended that it be hypercaloric and rich in fiber.

Conflict of interest

The authors declare no conflict of interest.

Author details

Maria Argente-Pla*, Katherine Garcia-Malpartida, Andrea Micó-García, Silvia Martín-Sanchis and Juan Francisco Merino-Torres
Endocrinology and Nutrition Department, La Fe Universitary Hospital, Valencia, Spain

*Address all correspondence to: mariaargentepla@gmail.com

References

[1] EFNS Task Force on Diagnosis and Management of Amyotrophic Lateral Sclerosis, Andersen PM, Abrahams S, Borasio GD, de Carvalho M, Chio A, et al. EFNS guidelines on the clinical management of amyotrophic lateral sclerosis (MALS)--revised report of an EFNS task force. European Journal of Neurology. 2012;**19**(3):360-375. DOI: 10.1111/j.1468-1331.2011.03501.x

[2] Logroscino G, Traynor BJ, Hardiman O, Chiò A, Mitchell D, Swingler RJ, et al. Incidence of amyotrophic lateral sclerosis in Europe. Journal of Neurology, Neurosurgery, and Psychiatry. 2010;**81**(4):385-390. DOI: 10.1136/jnnp.2009.183525

[3] Mehta P, Kaye W, Raymond J, Punjani R, Larson T, Cohen J, et al. Prevalence of amyotrophic lateral sclerosis - United States, 2015. MMWR. Morbidity and Mortality Weekly Report. 2018;**67**:1285-1289. DOI: 10.15585/mmwr.mm6746a1

[4] de Carvalho M, Dengler R, Eisen A, England JD, Kaji R, Kimura J, et al. Electrodiagnostic criteria for diagnosis of ALS. Clinical Neurophysiology. 2008;**119**:497-503. DOI: 10.1016/j.clinph.2007.09.143

[5] Brooks BR, Miller RG, Swash M, Munsat TL, World Federation of Neurology Research Group on Motor Neuron Diseases. El Escorial revisited: Revised criteria for the diagnosis of amyotrophic lateral sclerosis. Amyotrophic Lateral Sclerosis and Other Motor Neuron Disorders. 2000;**1**:293-299. DOI: 10.1080/146608200300079536

[6] Shefner JM, Al-Chalabi A, Baker MR, Cui LY, de Carvalho M, Eisen A, et al. A proposal for new diagnostic criteria for ALS. Clinical Neurophysiology. 2020;**131**(8):1975-1978. DOI: 10.1016/j.clinph.2020.04.005

[7] Ruoppolo G, Schettino I, Frasca V, Giacomelli E, Prosperini L, Cambieri C, et al. Dysphagia in amyotrophic lateral sclerosis: Prevalence and clinical findings. Acta Neurologica Scandinavica. 2013;**128**:397-401. DOI: 10.1111/ane.12136

[8] Miller RG, Mitchell JD, Moore DH. Riluzole for amyotrophic lateral sclerosis (ALS)/motor neuron disease (MND). Cochrane Database of Systematic Reviews. 2007;**24**(1):CD001447

[9] Hinchcliffe M, Smith A. Riluzole: Real-world evidence supports significant extension of median survival times in patients with amyotrophic lateral sclerosis. Degenerative Neurological and Neuromuscular Disease. 2017;**7**:61-70. DOI: 10.2147/DNND.S135748

[10] Worms PM. The epidemiology of motor neuron diseases: A review of recent studies. Journal of the Neurological Sciences. 2001;**191**:3-9. DOI: 10.1016/s0022-510x(01)00630-x

[11] Chiò A, Logroscino G, Hardiman O, Swingler R, Mitchell D, Beghi E, et al. Prognostic factors in ALS: A critical review. Amyotrophic Lateral Sclerosis. 2009;**10**:310-323. DOI: 10.3109/17482960802566824

[12] Burgos R, Bretón I, Cereda E, Desport JC, Dziewas R, Genton L, et al. ESPEN guideline clinical nutrition in neurology. Clinical Nutrition. 2018;**37**(1):354-396. DOI: 10.1016/j.clnu.2017.09.003

[13] Burkhardt C, Neuwirth C, Sommacal A, Andersen PM, Weber M. Is survival improved by the use of NIV and PEG in amyotrophic lateral sclerosis (ALS)? A post-mortem study of 80 ALS patients. PLoS One. 2017;**12**(5):e0177555. DOI: 10.1371/journal.pone.0177555

[14] Desport JC, Preux PM, Truong TC, Vallat JM, Sautereau D, Couratier P. Nutritional status is a prognostic factor for survival in ALS patients. Neurology. 1999;**53**(5):1059-1063. DOI: 10.1212/wnl.53.5.1059

[15] Virgili N. Soporte nutricional en el paciente con esclerosis lateral amiotrófica. InfoGeriatría. 2014;**10**:9-19

[16] Schindler JS, Kelly JH. Swallowing disorders in the elderly. The Laryngoscope. 2002;**112**(4):589-602. DOI: 10.1097/00005537-200204000-00001

[17] Mariani L, Ruoppolo G, Cilfone A, Cocchi C, Preziosi Standoli J, Longo L, et al. Progression of oropharyngeal dysphagia in amyotrophic lateral sclerosis: A retrospective Cohort Study. Dysphagia. DOI: 10.1007/s00455-021-10346-9

[18] Perry BJ, Stipancic KL, Martino R, Plowman EK, Green JR. Biomechanical biomarkers of tongue impairment during swallowing in persons diagnosed with amyotrophic lateral sclerosis. Dysphagia. 2021;**36**(1):147-156. DOI: 10.1007/s00455-020-10116-z

[19] Gwak DW, Jung SH, Min YS, Park JS, Cho HJ, Park D, et al. Correlation between maximal tongue pressure and swallowing function in spinal and bulbar muscular atrophy. Frontiers in Neurology. 2021;**12**:704788. DOI: 10.3389/fneur.2021.704788

[20] Yeates EM, Molfenter SM, Steele CM. Improvements in tongue strength and pressure-generation precision following a tongue pressure training protocol in older individuals with dysphagia: Three case reports. Clinical Interventions in Aging. 2008;**3**:735-747. DOI: 10.2147/cia.s3825

[21] Plowman EK, Watts SA, Robison R, Tabor L, Dion C, Gaziano J, et al. Voluntary cough airflow differentiates safe versus unsafe swallowing in amyotrophic lateral sclerosis. Dysphagia. 2016;**31**(3):383-390. DOI: 10.1007/s00455-015-9687-1

[22] Ertekin C, Aydogdu I, Yüceyar N, Kiylioglu N, Tarlaci S, Uludag B. Pathophysiological mechanisms of oropharyngeal dysphagia in amyotrophic lateral sclerosis. Brain. 2000;**123**:125-140. DOI: 10.1093/brain/123.1.125

[23] Tomik J, Sowula K, Dworak M, Stolcman K, Maraj M, Ceranowicz P. Esophageal peristalsis disorders in ALS patients with dysphagia. Brain Sciences. 2020;**10**(11):820. DOI: 10.3390/brainsci10110820

[24] Lee J, Madhavan A, Krajewski E, Lingenfelter S. Assessment of dysarthria and dysphagia in patients with amyotrophic lateral sclerosis: Review of the current evidence. Muscle & Nerve. 2021;**64**(5):520-531. DOI: 10.1002/mus.27361

[25] Tabor L, Gaziano J, Watts S, Robison R, Plowman EK. Defining swallowing-related quality of life profiles in individuals with amyotrophic lateral sclerosis. Dysphagia. 2016;**31**(3):376-382. DOI: 10.1007/s00455-015-9686-2

[26] Pattee GL, Plowman EK, Focht Garand KL, Costello J, Brooks BR, Berry JD, et al. Provisional best practices guidelines for the evaluation of bulbar dysfunction in amyotrophic lateral sclerosis. Muscle & Nerve. 2019;**59**(5):531-536. DOI: 10.1002/mus.26408

[27] Plowman EK, Tabor LC, Robison R, Gaziano J, Dion C, Watts SA, et al. Discriminant ability of the Eating Assessment Tool-10 to detect aspiration in individuals with amyotrophic lateral sclerosis. Neurogastroenterology and Motility. 2016;**28**(1):85-90. DOI: 10.1111/nmo.12700

[28] Higo R, Tayama N, Nito T. Longitudinal analysis of progression of dysphagia in amyotrophic lateral sclerosis. Auris, Nasus, Larynx. 2004;**31**:247-254. DOI: 10.1016/j.anl.2004.05.009

[29] Suiter DM, Sloggy J, Leder SB. Validation of the Yale swallow protocol: A prospective double-blinded videofluoroscopic study. Dysphagia. 2014;**29**:199-203. DOI: 10.1007/s00455-013-9488-3

[30] Aydougdu I, Zeynep Tanriverdi CE. Dysfunction of bulbar central pattern generator in ALS patients with dysphagia during sequential deglutition. Clinical Neurophysiology. 2011; **122**:1219-1228. DOI: 10.1016/j.clinph.2010.11.002

[31] Gaziano J, Tabor L, Richter J, Plowman E. Prevalence, Timing and Source of Aspiration in Individuals with ALS. Dysphagia Research Society. 2015.

[32] Kim J, Oh BM, Kim JY, Lee GJ, Lee SA, Han TR. Validation of the videofluoroscopic dysphagia scale in various etiologies. Dysphagia. 2014;**29**(4):438-443. DOI: 10.1007/s00455-014-9524-y

[33] Lee BJ, Eo H, Park D. Usefulness of the modified videofluoroscopic dysphagia scale in evaluating swallowing function among patients with amyotrophic lateral sclerosis and dysphagia. Journal of Clinical Medicine. 2021;**10**(19):4300. DOI: 10.3390/jcm10194300

[34] Fattori B, Siciliano G, Mancini V, Bastiani L, Bongioanni P, Caldarazzo Ienco E, et al. Dysphagia in amyotrophic lateral sclerosis: Relationships between disease progression and fiberoptic endoscopic evaluation of swallowing. Auris, Nasus, Larynx. 2017;**44**(3):306-312. DOI: 10.1016/j.anl.2016.07.002

[35] Pikus L, Levine MS, Yang YX, Rubesin SE, Katzka DA, Laufer I, et al. Videofluoroscopic studies of swallowing dysfunction and the relative risk of pneumonia. AJR. American Journal of Roentgenology. 2003;**180**(6):1613-1616. DOI: 10.2214/ajr.180.6.1801613

[36] DePaul R, Brooks BR. Multiple orofacial indices in amyotrophic lateral sclerosis. Journal of Speech, Language, and Hearing Research. 1993;**36**:1158-1167. DOI: 10.1044/jshr.3606.1158

[37] Weikamp JG, Schelhaas HJ, Hendriks JCM, de Swart BJM, Geurts ACH. Prognostic value of decreased tongue strength on survival time in patients with amyotrophic lateral sclerosis. Journal of Neurology. 2012;**259**:2360-2365. DOI: 10.1007/s00415-012-6503-9

[38] Hiraoka A, Yoshikawa M, Nakamori M, Hosomi N, Nagasaki T, Mori T, et al. Maximum tongue pressure is associated with swallowing dysfunction in ALS patients. Dysphagia. Aug 2017;**32**(4):542-547. DOI: 10.1007/s00455-017-9797-z

[39] Mann G. MASA: The Mann Assessment of Swallowing Ability. Clifton (NY): Tomson Learning Inc; 2002

[40] Plowman EK, Tabor LC, Wymer J, Pattee G. The evaluation of bulbar dysfunction in amyotrophic lateral sclerosis: Survey of clinical practice patterns in the United States. Amyotroph Lateral Scler Frontotemporal Degener. 2017;**18**:351-357. DOI: 10.1080/21678421.2017.1313868

[41] Epps D, Kwan JY, Russell JW, Thomas T, Diaz-Abad M. Evaluation and management of dysphagia in amyotrophic lateral sclerosis: a survey of speech-language pathologists' clinical practice. Journal of Clinical Neuromuscular Disease. 2020;**21**:135-143. DOI: 10.1097/CND.0000000000000281

[42] García-Peris P, Velasco C, Frías SL. Papel del equipo nutricional en el abordaje de la disfagia [Role of the nutritional support team in the management of dysphagia]. Nutrición Hospitalaria. 2014;**29**(Suppl 2):13-21 Spanish

[43] Solazzo A, Del Vecchio L, Reginelli A, Monaco L, Sagnelli A, Monsorrò M, et al. Search for compensation postures with videofluoromanometric investigation in dysphagic patients affected by amyotrophic lateral sclerosis. La Radiologia Medica. 2011;**116**(7):1083-1094. DOI: 10.1007/s11547-011-0698-1

[44] Greenwood DI. Nutrition management of amyotrophic lateral sclerosis. Nutrition in Clinical Practice. 2013;**28**(3):392-399. DOI: 10.1177/0884533613476554

[45] Trumbo P, Schlicker S, Yates AA, Poos M, Food and Nutrition Board of the Institute of Medicine, The National Academies. Dietary reference intakes for energy, carbohydrate, fiber, fat, fatty acids, cholesterol, protein and amino acids. Journal of the American Dietetic Association. 2002;**102**(11):1621-1630. DOI: 10.1016/s0002-8223(02)90346-9

[46] Institute of Medicine (US) Committee to Review Dietary Reference Intakes for Vitamin D and Calcium. Dietary Reference Intakes for Calcium and Vitamin D. Ross AC, Taylor CL, Yaktine AL, Del Valle HB, editors. Washington (DC): National Academies Press (US); 2011. DOI:10.17226/13050

[47] Institute of Medicine (US) Standing Committee on the Scientific Evaluation of Dietary Reference Intakes. Dietary Reference Intakes for Calcium, Phosphorus, Magnesium, Vitamin D, and Fluoride. Washington (DC): National Academies Press (US); 1997. DOI: 10.17226/5776

[48] Institute of Medicine (US) Standing Committee on the Scientific Evaluation of Dietary Reference Intakes and its Panel on Folate, Other B Vitamins, and Choline. Dietary Reference Intakes for Thiamin, Riboflavin, Niacin, Vitamin B6, Folate, Vitamin B12, Pantothenic Acid, Biotin, and Choline. Washington (DC): National Academies Press (US); 1998. DOI: 10.17226/6015

[49] Institute of Medicine (US) Panel on Dietary Antioxidants and Related Compounds. Dietary Reference Intakes for Vitamin C, Vitamin E, Selenium, and Carotenoids. Washington (DC): National Academies Press (US); 2000. DOI: 10.17226/9810

[50] Institute of Medicine (US) Panel on Micronutrients. Dietary Reference Intakes for Vitamin A, Vitamin K, Arsenic, Boron, Chromium, Copper, Iodine, Iron, Manganese, Molybdenum, Nickel, Silicon, Vanadium, and Zinc. Washington (DC): National Academies Press (US); 2001. DOI: 10.17226/10026

[51] Cichero JA, Lam P, Steele CM, Hanson B, Chen J, Dantas RO, et al. Development of international terminology and definitions for texture-modified foods and thickened fluids used in dysphagia management: The IDDSI framework. Dysphagia. 2017;**32**(2):293-314. DOI: 10.1007/s00455-016-9758-y

[52] Garcia JM, Chambers E 4th, Matta Z, Clark M. Viscosity measurements of nectar- and honey-thick liquids: product, liquid, and time comparisons. Dysphagia. 2005;**20**(4):325-335. DOI: 10.1007/s00455-005-0034-9

[53] Carbó Perseguer J, Madejón Seiz A, Romero Portales M, Martínez Hernández J, Mora Pardina JS, García-Samaniego J. Percutaneous endoscopic gastrostomy in patients with amyotrophic lateral sclerosis: Mortality and complications. Neurologia (Engl Ed). 2019;**34**(9):582-588. DOI: 10.1016/j.nrl.2018.01.003

[54] Miller RG, Jackson CE, Kasarskis EJ, England JD, Forshew D, Johnston W, et al. Practice parameter update: The care of the patient with amyotrophic lateral sclerosis: Drug, nutritional, and respiratory therapies (an evidence-based review): Report of the Quality Standards Subcommittee of the American Academy of Neurology. Neurology. 2009;**73**(15):1218-1226. DOI: 10.1212/WNL.0b013e3181bc0141

[55] Pena MJ, Ravasco P, Machado M, Pinto A, Pinto S, Rocha L, et al. What is the relevance of percutaneous endoscopic gastrostomy on the survival of patients with amyotrophic lateral sclerosis? Amyotrophic Lateral Sclerosis. 2012;**13**(6):550-554. DOI: 10.3109/17482968.2012.684215

[56] Sarfaty M, Nefussy B, Gross D, Shapira Y, Vaisman N, Drory VE. Outcome of percutaneous endoscopic gastrostomy insertion in patients with amyotrophic lateral sclerosis in relation to respiratory dysfunction. Amyotroph Lateral Scler Frontotemporal Degener. 2013;**14**(7-8):528-532. DOI: 10.3109/21678421.2013.812659

[57] Spataro R, Ficano L, Piccoli F, La Bella V. Percutaneous endoscopic gastrostomy in amyotrophic lateral sclerosis: effect on survival. Journal of the Neurological Sciences. 2011;**304**(1-2): 44-48. DOI: 10.1016/j.jns.2011.02.016

[58] Jiménez García I, Sala Moya N, Riera Munt M, Herrera Rodríguez MV, Povedano Panadés M, Virgili Casas MN. La opinión del paciente cuenta: Experiencia en la atención nutricional en un equipo multidisciplinar de ELA [The patient's opinion matters: experience in the nutritional care in an ALS multidisciplinary team]. Nutrición Hospitalaria. 2015;**31**(Suppl 5):56-66. Spanish. DOI: 10.3305/nh.2015.31.sup5.9132

[59] López-Gómez JJ, Ballesteros-Pomar MD, Torres-Torres B, Pintor-De la Maza B, Penacho-Lázaro MA, Palacio-Mures JM, et al. Impact of percutaneous endoscopic gastrostomy (PEG) on the evolution of disease in patients with amyotrophic lateral sclerosis (ALS). Nutrients. 2021;**13**(8): 2765. DOI: 10.3390/nu13082765

Chapter 3

Dysphagia in Neuroinflammatory Diseases of the Central Nervous System

Fereshteh Ghadiri and Abdorreza Naser Moghadasi

Abstract

Neuroinflammatory disorders of the central nervous system (CNS) consist of a relatively heterogeneous group of diseases that share the autoimmune activity against different parts of the system. Swallowing problems could happen in many of these cases. Its effect on the patients' quality of life is undeniable. It could be an important cause of morbidity and mortality. Detailed medical history and physical exam are important. Several questionnaires could help monitor dysphagia. Radiographic and endoscopic evaluations may be necessary to detect overlooked swallowing problems. The main treatment appears to be treating the underlying disease, besides general supplementary options like rehabilitation and speech therapy.

Keywords: dysphagia, inflammation, central nervous system, multiple sclerosis, neuromyelitis optica

1. Introduction

Dysphagia, as described in different sections of this book, is referred to as any difficulty in swallowing and deglutition. It could happen in the oral, pharyngeal, or esophageal phases. Any disturbance from the cortex to the involved muscle could interfere with easy and successful swallowing.

Neuroinflammatory disorders of the central nervous system (CNS) consist of a relatively heterogeneous group of diseases that share the autoimmune activity against different parts of the system. The trigger is not clearly determined, but a wide range of genetic and environmental factors are suggested. Both cellular and humoral immune responses could be affected. Each disease in this category has a predilection to specific areas of the CNS. However, exceptions are not rare and generally, any part of the CNS could get involved. This variability results in miscellaneous presentations. Swallowing problems could happen in many of these cases. This could be due to lesions in the cortex affecting deglutition muscles, sensory pathway disturbance, or impaired swallowing reflexes. Cognitive dysfunction may further complicate the situation. Its effect on the patients' quality of life is undeniable. It could be an important cause of morbidity and mortality (**Table 1**).

In this chapter, we will review this underestimated but still an important cause of deglutition problems.

IntechOpen

Multiple sclerosis *Neuromyelitis optica spectrum disease* *Myelin oligodendrocyte glycoprotein antibody disease (MOGAD)* *Autoimmune encephalitis* • Anti IgLON5 • DPPX potassium channel antibody • Anti-Ma2 • Hashimoto encephalitis • Anti-Neuronal Nuclear Autoantibody Type 2 (ANNA-2) or "anti-Ri" • Autoimmune glial fibrillary acidic protein (GFAP) astrocytopathy • Anti-neurochondrin • Bickerstaff's brainstem encephalitis • Acute disseminated encephalomyelitis (ADEM) • Chronic lymphocytic inflammation with pontine perivascular enhancement responsive to steroids (CLIPPERS) *Systemic autoimmune disorders with CNS involvement* • Behcet's disease • Systematic lupus erythematous • Sjogren syndrome • Sarcoidosis

Table 1.
Inflammatory diseases of the CNS with dysphagia.

2. Multiple sclerosis

Multiple sclerosis (MS) is the most popular autoimmune disorder of the CNS. Its prevalence may range from 2 to 100 per 100,000 in different areas of the world [1] but its incidence is absolutely rising [2]. The disease could involve any part of the CNS, leading to its wide range of manifestations. The course may be relapsing-remitting or progressive. The disability is estimated via measures like the expanded disability status scale (EDSS) or patient-determined disease steps (PDDS) [3].

Acute or chronic demyelinating lesions in related cortical areas, sensorimotor pathways, and balance systems could lead to various difficulties in swallowing. Kapitza et al. also have discussed the potential role of esophageal glial cells [4]. The first reports of these symptoms go back to 1877 but it still is underestimated [5]. Dysphagia to liquids seems to be as prevalent as solid food swallowing difficulty in MS [6]. This could significantly impact the patients' quality of life [7], putting them in danger of malnutrition [8], even fatal aspiration pneumonia. The latter is the leading cause of death in MS [9]. Silent aspiration is also common (40%) [10].

2.1 Epidemiology

Dysphagia is notably prevalent among these patients. It seems to affect at least over 30% of the MS population [5]. Besides, objective examinations may find the problem in as high as 80% of the cases [5, 11]. It highlights the issue of underreporting this symptom and the importance of detailed clinical evaluation and using more advanced diagnostic tools, especially in high-risk cases [12].

On the other hand, there is a considerable discrepancy between reports from different regions. Based on a systematic review in 2015, Iran has the lowest and Europe has the highest reported prevalence of dysphagia in MS [5].

As predicted, those with higher disability scores and longer duration of disease are at more risk of experiencing deglutition difficulties [5, 11, 13, 14].

Nonetheless, it is not rare in earlier stages of the disease [14]. It could be mild and intermittent or severe and disabling. In a study from Brazil, of 108 MS patients, 90% showed different stages of dysphagia. Most cases showed mild to moderate degrees of difficulty. About 12.5% had severe dysphagia, most of whom were in progressive stages of MS and had higher EDSS [11].

2.2 Pathophysiology

Brainstem and cerebellar lesions appear to be more associated with dysphagia [13, 15]. Pharyngeal phase is more likely to be involved [13]. This could be the consequence of impaired gag reflex or uncoordinated muscle contractions [12].

To name some other pathologies that interfere with successful swallowing, we could mention cranial neuralgias and facial paresis. Cranial (trigeminal, glossopharyngeal, or occipital) neuralgias could happen in MS. These painful electric-shock like attacks could alter easy swallowing in different phases, dependent on the involved area. Disturbed sensation may further complicate the process. Facial paresis could be another intervening problem. It may result in inadequate chewing that would make the bolus hard to swallow. In addition, cognitive impairment could exaggerate the problem.

2.3 Screening with questionnaires

DYMUS (DYsphagia in MUltiple Sclerosis) was developed to screen MS patients for self-reported dysphagia in 2008 [16]. It is a self-assessment tool with 10 yes or no questions. Several studies evaluated the original and translated versions [17–20]. The modified version was introduced in 2020. It has shown to improve the psychometric properties of DYMUS [21]. Other less specific-to-MS questionnaires include the Eating Assessment Tool (EAT), the Swallowing Quality of Life (SWAL-QoL). EAT consists of 10 questions that provide information about functional, physical, and emotional consequences of dysphagia. It is not a time-consuming test, while 44 questions of SWAL-QoL may be considered as an important limitation. The Yale Swallow Protocol, the Gugging Swallowing Screen, and the Test of Masticating and Swallowing Solids have also been used [12]. As mentioned before, relying only on the self-reported symptoms could underestimate the problem so more in-depth clinical and paraclinical assessments may be essential. Still, patient-reported assessments may give a better picture of the psychosocial burden of the problem [16].

2.4 Clinical assessment

Paying attention to the drugs that may cause oral side effects including dysphagia should be in mind. Glatiramer acetate is a disease-modifying drug that could cause dysphagia. Anticonvulsants like clonazepam are reported to have this adverse effect. Oxybutynin, a commonly used treatment for bladder symptoms of MS, is another accusable medication. Amantadine as a fatigue treatment and dantrolene as a spasmolytic agent could also alter deglutition [17].

Apart from the standard neurological examination (mental state, cranial nerves, motor forces, sensory system, reflexes, coordination, and gait), some clues could be of help, especially for detecting unreported aspiration. For instance, dysarthria could be an indicator of concomitant dysphagia [18]. Another indicator could be coughing or choking during meal [14]. Three-ounce (90 cc) water swallowing test, although not yet validated in MS, is a sensitive tool to identify those at risk of aspiration [19]. Some authorities recommend regular evaluations by otolaryngologists in high-risk patients [20].

Electrophysiologic methods could detect subclinical dysphagia [21, 22]. Fiberoptic endoscopic evaluation of swallowing (FEES) [23] and videofluoroscopic study of swallowing (VFSS) also seem reliable techniques [22]. FEES is a flexible endoscope introduced in 1988. It is inserted through the nose and investigates laryngeal and pharyngeal functions [24]. Grading scores show the severity of dysphagia. Some recommended this method as a standard screening method in older patients with advanced stages of MS [23]. VFSS assesses the oral, pharyngeal, laryngeal, and upper esophageal phases after ingestion of barium-containing material, in a seated position. In a study by Wiesner et al., of eight patients without any subjective complaint, only two had normal VFSS [25]. MS could result in delayed pharyngeal phase, shorter laryngeal excursion, and longer intervals between airway closure and upper esophageal sphincter opening [26].

The diagnostic steps are summarized in **Table 2**.

2.5 Treatment

The first important step to take, after stabilization of the patient, is to determine if the dysphagia is a consequence of an acute attack or not (the other differentials could be pseudo relapse due to infections, progression of previously encountered mild dysphagia, medication adverse events, local pathologies of the gastrointestinal tract, or another disease like Guillain-Barre syndrome, botulism, myasthenia gravis or many other diseases). If the relapse is proven, anti-inflammatory treatments of acute relapse may be helpful to alleviate the symptom. These treatments include steroids, intravenous immunoglobulins (IVIg), and plasma exchange in refractory cases. The treatment choice would depend on the patient's condition, contraindications for receiving any of the aforementioned options, and the availability of the treatment. The next step is to decide if the disease-modifying treatment should be switched, or started in a treatment-naïve patient.

Medical history • Dysphagia clues: "coughing" or "choking" during meals, dysarthria • Onset, progression, associated symptoms • Medications: Glatiramer acetate, anticonvulsants like clonazepam, oxybutynin, dantrolene • Weight loss, symptoms of malnutrition • Symptoms of aspiration
Further evaluation: • Questionnaires: DYMUS, EAT, SWAL-QoL, the Yale Swallow Protocol, the Gugging Swallowing Screen, Test of Masticating and Swallowing Solids • Three-ounce (90 cc) water swallowing test • Thorough neurologic exam • Systemic physical exam • FEES • VFSS • Consults with otolaryngologist, or gastroenterologist as indicated
DYMUS: DYsphagia in MUltiple Sclerosis, EAT: Eating Assessment Tool, SWAL-QoL: Swallowing Quality of Life, FEES: fiberoptic endoscopic evaluation of swallowing, VFSS: videofluoroscopic study of swallowing.

Table 2.
Approach to dysphagia in MS.

Apart from the initial immune therapy, an integrated multidisciplinary approach is needed to see the patients' needs. Neurologists, dentists, and otolaryngologists should be informed about the subject. Speech therapists [27] and dieticians could be of great help. Lifestyle modifications (finding the best head, neck, and chest position, the most proper food consistency [28], oral hygiene) and investigation for possible guilty medication could be the first steps to take. Electrical stimulation [29, 30] and botulinum toxin injection are the two most studied treatments for dysphagia in MS [31]. Botulinum toxin is suitable when there are signs of the hyperactive sphincter (cricopharyngeal muscle) [32]. It should be performed by experienced hands to avert the possible adverse effects [31, 33]. The evidence on electrical stimulation is still not sufficient but some promising effects have been seen [30, 34, 35]. Marrosu et al. suggested that this modulation of central pattern generators of swallowing via vagus nerve stimulation could have positive effects [29].

Gastrostomy is the final solution in advanced cases. It has been shown that more than 50% of MS patients with gastrostomy lived two or more years after the procedure [36].

Transcranial direct current stimulation is another investigatory method with initial positive results [37, 38].

Cognitive rehabilitation could be a useful strategy to tackle the associated problems that may worsen the swallowing problems [39].

3. Neuromyelitis optica spectrum disorder (NMOSD)

Neuromyelitis optica spectrum disorders (NMOSD) is another member of the neuroinflammatory diseases category. Compared with MS, it is more of an antibody-based astrocytopathy. The guilt is on antiaquaporine4, an autoantibody against water channels that are mostly found in special areas of the CNS. This nonprogressive, relapsing condition could trigger necrotizing attacks on the brain, optic nerves, or spinal cord. Brainstem involvement is common. Therefore, deglutition difficulties are expected, but it seems to be rare.

Dysphagia in these patients could be the manifestation of an acute attack, and even the presenting symptom [40, 41]. It is significantly associated with lesions in the brainstem and specially medulla oblongata. In a study by Wang et al. of 170 NMOSD patients, 15 experienced dysphagia most of whom had medullary lesions. It is speculated that involvement of nucleus ambiguous, nucleus tractus solitarius, or dorsal vagus nucleus may be responsible [42]. It also can be a sign of cerebral involvement in the absence of other evidence [43, 44]. In seven NMO patients reported by Pawlitzki et al., five showed degrees of dysphagia, mostly mild to moderate. All had brainstem or high cervical lesions. Here again, FEES could be of great help in diagnosing subtle cases [43]. As in MS, NMO cases with dysphagia have problems with swallowing both solid food and liquids [6].

The fundamentals of diagnosis and treatment of dysphagia in this population are like MS. However, as the attacks are necrotizing, no time should be lost before initiating immune therapy. The only available disease-modifying treatments in NMOSD are anti CD20s (rituximab, satralizumab, eculizumab). The chosen option should be started as soon as possible after initial relapse treatment.

4. Myelin oligodendrocyte glycoprotein antibody disease (MOGAD)

Another autoimmune demyelinating disease is MOGAD. The antibody was discovered about 40 years ago [45] but its clinical relevance was found years later [46]. There are doubts about the pathogenicity of the anti-MOG antibody but still, it is the best available biomarker of the disease to date [47]. The clinical manifestations of MOGAD overlap with NMOSD (optic neuritis, spinal lesion, brainstem involvement), although with some differences. Cortical lesions are more prevalent in MOGAD. Astrocytes are hypertrophic and reactive, not dystrophic compared with NMOSD. Besides, there is no aquaporin4 loss [47]. Acute disseminated encephalomyelitis (ADEM) like presentation is common among children with the disease [48]. It could be monophasic (70–80% in children) or relapsing. In monophasic cases, the antibody tends to become undetectable over 12 months, so follow-up is recommended [47]. The mainstay of the treatment is anti-inflammatory drugs like steroids in the acute phase and anti CD20s as maintenance treatment.

As a rare entity, there are not many reports on specific symptoms like swallowing difficulties. However, considering the CNS involvement (especially with cortical and brainstem lesions) dysphagia is expected. Of 50 patients in a European cohort of Caucasian MOGAD cases, 15 had brainstem involvement. Of these only two complained of dysphagia besides other symptoms [49]. As in NMOSD, brain involvement in MOGAD may only present with dysphagia detected by FEES [43].

5. Autoimmune encephalitis

This category consists of heterogeneous conditions; all share the feature of autoimmunity against different components of the CNS. The antibodies may target against intraneural or cell surface molecules (synaptic receptors, ion channels, other molecules). They may be accompanied by an underlying neoplasm. Experts recommend to have this diagnosis in mind whenever facing a subacute encephalopathy with focal neurologic findings (clinically or in imaging) [50]. Dysphagia is reported in various subtypes of the disease.

Anti IgLON5 disease is a relatively novel entity characterized by sleep-related diseases like REM or non-REM parasomnias, obstructive sleep apnea, and stridor. This disease may present similar to neurodegenerative diseases. It is progressive and could be fatal (e.g. due to central hypoventilation). By early diagnosis and treatment, there is hope in halting the disease's progression to respiratory arrest. Bulbar symptoms are quite prevalent. Dysphagia is the most common bulbar symptom in this population. Other manifestations include gait instability, dysautonomia, movement disorders, supranuclear gaze palsy, and cognitive impairment [51, 52].

In a case series of 20 patients with DPPX potassium channel antibody, 15 had brainstem involvement of whom six patients experienced dysphagia along with other symptoms. DPPX potassium channel antibody is "immunoglobulin G (IgG) targeting dipeptidyl-peptidase-like protein-6 (DPPX), a regulatory subunit of neuronal Kv4.2 potassium channels" [53].

Castle et al. reported a 39-year-old patient who presented with subacute progressive behavioral changes, dysphagia, and ataxia. Anti-Ma2 was detected and cancer work-up revealed metastatic testicular cancer. Anti-Ma2 encephalitis involves the brainstem commonly. Dysphagia is present in 20% of these cases [54].

A 14-year-old boy has been reported who had dysphagia, unilateral weakness, and aggressiveness as presenting symptoms of autoimmune encephalitis caused by Hashimoto disease. The point is that the patient had no previous clinical clue of thyroiditis. Hashimoto encephalitis could manifest with a variety of clinical scenarios so it should be in mind whenever facing an autoimmune pathology of the CNS [55].

Anti-Neuronal Nuclear Autoantibody Type 2 (ANNA-2) or "anti-Ri" is an uncommon antibody detected among cases of paraneoplastic encephalitis. It could be associated with several underlying cancers. Pittock et al. detected this marker in 34 patients in 75,000 patients with suspected paraneoplastic neurologic symptoms. Brainstem symptoms including dysphagia were prevalent among these cases. Involvement of other parts of the nervous system (cortex, basal ganglia, cerebellum, spinal cord, cranial nerves, peripheral nerves, or neuromuscular junction) was also seen [56].

Autoimmune glial fibrillary acidic protein (GFAP) astrocytopathy is a recently introduced disease. The inflammation in this disease involves meninges in addition to other parts of the CNS. It could cause headache, visual disturbance, fever, psychosis, myelitis, ataxia, abnormal movements, or autonomic dysfunction. The MRI would show linear enhancement oriented radially to the ventricles in the brain. A reported case by Li et al. highlights the possibility of dysphagia being a part of the initial presentation [57].

Dysphagia, albeit not common, could also be seen in those with IgG autoantibody targeted against neuronal cytosolic protein, neurochondrin. These cases mostly present with cerebellar symptoms [58]. Likewise, dysphagia is described in association with anti-Ca, an established cause of cerebellar ataxia [59].

Bickerstaff's brainstem encephalitis overlaps with Guillain-Barre and Miller-Fisher diseases. Around 40—60% of cases may have anti-GQ1b IgG in their serum [60]. In the earliest report, six of seven cases had complete bulbar paralysis. However, milder degrees of dysphagia may be present and overlooked, as one case of silent aspiration is reported. Dietrich-Burns et al. emphasize to be aware of this issue as cognitive impairment may lead to underreporting [61].

There are other conditions with less known underlying autoantibodies. Acute disseminated encephalomyelitis (ADEM) is a mostly monophasic disease, more common among children, that can present with a broad spectrum of symptoms. Dysphagia has been reported as the sole manifestation of the disease in some cases [62]. Although as mentioned earlier, some cases may be anti MOG positive. Furthermore, chronic lymphocytic inflammation with pontine perivascular enhancement responsive to steroids (CLIPPERS) is another similar entity with specific clinical and imaging characteristics. As the main site of involvement is the brainstem, dysphagia could happen in the course of the disease [63].

6. Systemic autoimmune disorders

Last but not the least are systemic autoimmune diseases that can involve CNS variably. They include Behcet's disease, systematic lupus erythematosus (SLE), Sjogren syndrome, and sarcoidosis.

6.1 Behcet's disease

Initially described in 1937, the disease is well known for causing oral and genital aphthous lesions, along with uveitis. Gradually, it became clear that the patients may experience ulcerations in other parts of the gastrointestinal tract, like esophagus [64]. But this local pathology is not the sole cause of dysphagia in this disease. CNS involvement in Behcet's disease is an established neuroinflammatory pathology. The parenchymal involvement has a significant predilection to the brainstem so dysphagia is expected. Vascular pathologies of the CNS could affect successful swallowing, as well [65, 66].

6.2 SLE

Global structural disintegration could occur in association with CNS involvement due to SLE [67]. Headache, seizure, psychiatric changes, and a wide range of other neurologic complaints could ensue [68]. Dysphagia in SLE is mostly the result of local pathologies (esophageal motility disorder, concomitant gastroesophageal reflux disorder, and esophagitis) [69], but with CNS involvement, neurogenic dysphagia is not unexpected.

6.3 Sjogren's syndrome

Xerostomia and xerophthalmia are hallmarks of the disease. Associated neuropathies [70], optic neuritis, and associated NMOSD [71] are reported. Gastrointestinal manifestations are diverse and various causes could be encountered; of which local pathologies dominate [72] (like SLE). However, CNS involvement should be in mind when facing difficult swallowing complaints.

6.4 Neurosarcoidosis

Sarcoidosis is known to cause noncaseating granulomata and mediastinal lymphadenopathy. Neurosarcoidosis may be present in 5–16% of cases. It could involve any part of the CNS. This differential should be considered whenever confronting inflammatory lesions of the nervous system. However, some symptoms are considered more specific to neurosarcoidosis like bifacial paresis (especially in the presence of uveitis and parotiditis), pituitary/hypothalamus lesions, longitudinally extensive myelitis, and cauda equina syndrome [73].

Deglutition problems are not frequent in sarcoidosis. The most common cause of dysphagia in these patients is the compressive effect of enlarged lymph nodes. Less commonly there is direct esophageal pathology. Neurosarcoidosis is a rare cause of dysphagia. Still, there are cases with dysphagia as a presenting symptom of the disease [74, 75].

7. Conclusions

Neuroinflammatory disorders of the CNS include a heterogeneous group that could interfere with successful swallowing. The associated dysphagia could be transitory or permanent depending on the pathology (transient inflammation versus necrosis). Detailed medical history and physical exam are the important assets of diagnosis. Several questionnaires could help monitor dysphagia. Radiographic and endoscopic evaluations may be necessary to detect overlooked swallowing problems. The main treatment appears to be treating the underlying disease, besides general supplementary options like rehabilitation and speech therapy.

Author details

Fereshteh Ghadiri and Abdorreza Naser Moghadasi*
Multiple Sclerosis Research Center, Neuroscience Institute, Tehran University of Medical Sciences, Tehran, Iran

*Address all correspondence to: abdorrezamoghadasi@gmail.com

References

[1] Howard J, Trevick S, Younger DS. Epidemiology of multiple sclerosis. Neurologic Clinics. 2016;**34**(4):919-939. DOI: 10.1016/j.ncl.2016.06.016

[2] Koch-Henriksen N, Magyari M. Apparent changes in the epidemiology and severity of multiple sclerosis. Nature Reviews Neurology. 2021;**17**(11): 676-688. DOI: 10.1038/s41582-021-00556-y

[3] Learmonth YC, Motl RW, Sandroff BM, Pula JH, Cadavid D. Validation of patient determined disease steps (PDDS) scale scores in persons with multiple sclerosis. BMC Neurology. 2013;**13**:37. DOI: 10.1186/1471-2377-13-37

[4] Kapitza C, Chunder R, Scheller A, Given KS, Macklin WB, Enders M, et al. Murine esophagus expresses glial-derived central nervous system antigens. International Journal of Molecular Sciences. 2021;**22**(6). DOI: 10.3390/ijms22063233

[5] Guan XL, Wang H, Huang HS, Meng L. Prevalence of dysphagia in multiple sclerosis: A systematic review and meta-analysis. Neurological Sciences. 2015;**36**(5):671-681. DOI: 10.1007/s10072-015-2067-7

[6] Milewska M, Grabarczyk K, Dabrowska-Bender M, et al. The prevalence and types of oral- and pharyngeal-stage dysphagia in patients with demyelinating diseases based on subjective assessment by the study subjects. Multiple Sclerosis and Related Disorders. 2020;**37**:101484. DOI: 10.1016/j.msard.2019.101484

[7] Tahir E, Kavaz E, Kemal O, Sen S, Terzi M. Screening of dysphagia by DYMUS (Dysphagia in multiple sclerosis) and SWAL-QoL (Swallowing quality of life) surveys in patients with multiple sclerosis. Multiple Sclerosis and Related Disorders. 2020;**45**:102397. DOI: 10.1016/j.msard.2020.102397

[8] Pasquinelli S, Solaro C. Nutritional assessment and malnutrition in multiple sclerosis. Neurological Sciences. 2008;**29**(Suppl. 4):S367-S369. DOI: 10.1007/s10072-008-1046-7

[9] Lunde HMB, Assmus J, Myhr KM, Bo L, Grytten N. Survival and cause of death in multiple sclerosis: A 60-year longitudinal population study. Journal of Neurology, Neurosurgery, and Psychiatry. 2017;**88**(8):621-625. DOI: 10.1136/jnnp-2016-315238

[10] Terre-Boliart R, Orient-Lopez F, Guevara-Espinosa D, Ramon-Rona S, Bernabeu-Guitart M, Clave-Civit P. Disfagia orofaringea en pacientes afectados de esclerosis multiple [Oropharyngeal dysphagia in patients with multiple sclerosis]. Revista de Neurologia. 2004;**39**(8):707-710

[11] Fernandes AM, Duprat Ade C, Eckley CA, Silva L, Ferreira RB, Tilbery CP. Oropharyngeal dysphagia in patients with multiple sclerosis: Do the disease classification scales reflect dysphagia severity? Brazilian Journal of Otorhinolaryngology. 2013;**79**(4):460-465. DOI: 10.5935/1808-8694.20130082

[12] De Biagi F, Heikkola LM, Nordio S, Ruhaak L. Update on recent developments in communication and swallowing in multiple sclerosis. International Journal of MS Care. 2020;**22**(6):270-275. DOI: 10.7224/1537-2073.2020-023

[13] Poorjavad M, Derakhshandeh F, Etemadifar M, Soleymani B, Minagar A, Maghzi AH. Oropharyngeal dysphagia in multiple sclerosis. Multiple Sclerosis. 2010;**16**(3):362-365. DOI: 10.1177/1352458509358089

[14] De Pauw A, Dejaeger E, D'Hooghe B, Carton H. Dysphagia in multiple sclerosis. Clinical Neurology and Neurosurgery. 2002;**104**(4):345-351. DOI: 10.1016/s0303-8467(02)00053-7

[15] Calcagno P, Ruoppolo G, Grasso MG, De Vincentiis M, Paolucci S. Dysphagia in multiple sclerosis—prevalence and prognostic factors. Acta Neurologica Scandinavica. 2002;**105**(1):40-43. DOI: 10.1034/j.1600-0404.2002.10062.x

[16] Keage M, Delatycki M, Corben L, Vogel A. A systematic review of self-reported swallowing assessments in progressive neurological disorders. Dysphagia. 2015;**30**(1):27-46. DOI: 10.1007/s00455-014-9579-9

[17] Cockburn N, Pateman K, Taing MW, Pradhan A, Ford PJ. Managing the oral side-effects of medications used to treat multiple sclerosis. Australian Dental Journal. 2017;**62**(3):331-336. DOI: 10.1111/adj.12510

[18] Wang BJ, Carter FL, Altman KW. Relationship between dysarthria and oral-oropharyngeal dysphagia: The current evidence. Ear Nose Throat Journal. 2018;**97**(3):E1-e9

[19] DePippo KL, Holas MA, Reding MJ. Validation of the 3-oz water swallow test for aspiration following stroke. Archives of Neurology. 1992;**49**(12):1259-1261. DOI: 10.1001/archneur.1992.005303 60057018

[20] Di Stadio A, Bernitsas E. Otolaryngological symptoms and multiple sclerosis: A forgotten and underestimated relationship. Multiple Sclerosis and Related Disorders. 2019;**28**:197-198. DOI: 10.1016/j.msard.2019.01.010

[21] Beckmann Y, Gurgor N, Cakir A, et al. Electrophysiological evaluation of dysphagia in the mild or moderate patients with multiple sclerosis: A concept of subclinical dysphagia. Dysphagia. 2015;**30**(3):296-303. DOI: 10.1007/s00455-015-9598-1

[22] Alfonsi E, Bergamaschi R, Cosentino G, et al. Electrophysiological patterns of oropharyngeal swallowing in multiple sclerosis. Clinical Neurophysiology. 2013;**124**(8):1638-1645. DOI: 10.1016/j.clinph.2013.03.003

[23] Solaro C, Cuccaro A, Gamberini G, et al. Prevalence of dysphagia in a consecutive cohort of subjects with MS using fibre-optic endoscopy. Neurological Sciences. 2020;**41**(5):1075-1079. DOI: 10.1007/s10072-019-04198-3

[24] Langmore SE, Schatz K, Olsen N. Fiberoptic endoscopic examination of swallowing safety: A new procedure. Dysphagia. 1988;**2**(4):216-219. DOI: 10.1007/BF02414429

[25] Wiesner W, Wetzel SG, Kappos L, et al. Swallowing abnormalities in multiple sclerosis: Correlation between videofluoroscopy and subjective symptoms. European Radiology. 2002;**12**(4):789-792. DOI: 10.1007/s003300101086

[26] Abraham SS, Yun PT. Laryngopharyngeal dysmotility in multiple sclerosis. Dysphagia. 2002;**17**(1):69-74. DOI: 10.1007/s00455-001-0103-7

[27] Tarameshlu M, Ghelichi L, Azimi AR, Ansari NN, Khatoonabadi AR. The effect of traditional dysphagia therapy on the swallowing function in patients with multiple sclerosis: A pilot double-blinded randomized controlled trial. Journal of Bodywork and Movement Therapies. 2019;**23**(1):171-176. DOI: 10.1016/j.jbmt.2018.01.016

[28] Giusti A, Giambuzzi M. Management of dysphagia in patients affected by multiple sclerosis: State of the art. Neurological Sciences. 2008;**29**(Suppl. 4):S364-S366. DOI: 10.1007/s10072-008-1045-8

[29] Marrosu F, Maleci A, Cocco E, Puligheddu M, Barberini L, Marrosu MG. Vagal nerve stimulation improves cerebellar tremor and

dysphagia in multiple sclerosis. Multiple Sclerosis. 2007;**13**(9):1200-1202. DOI: 10.1177/1352458507078399

[30] Bogaardt H, van Dam D, Wever NM, Bruggeman CE, Koops J, Fokkens WJ. Use of neuromuscular electrostimulation in the treatment of dysphagia in patients with multiple sclerosis. The Annals of Otology, Rhinology, and Laryngology. 2009;**118**(4):241-246. DOI: 10.1177/000348940911800401

[31] Alali D, Ballard K, Bogaardt H. Treatment effects for dysphagia in adults with multiple sclerosis: A systematic review. Dysphagia. 2016;**31**(5):610-618. DOI: 10.1007/s00455-016-9738-2

[32] Restivo DA, Marchese-Ragona R, Patti F, et al. Botulinum toxin improves dysphagia associated with multiple sclerosis. European Journal of Neurology. 2011;**18**(3):486-490. DOI: 10.1111/j.1468-1331.2010.03189.x

[33] Alfonsi E, Merlo IM, Ponzio M, et al. An electrophysiological approach to the diagnosis of neurogenic dysphagia: Implications for botulinum toxin treatment. Journal of Neurology, Neurosurgery, and Psychiatry. 2010;**81**(1):54-60. DOI: 10.1136/jnnp.2009.174698

[34] Restivo DA, Casabona A, Centonze D, Marchese-Ragona R, Maimone D, Pavone A. Pharyngeal electrical stimulation for dysphagia associated with multiple sclerosis: A pilot study. Brain Stimulation. 2013;**6**(3):418-423. DOI: 10.1016/j.brs.2012.09.001

[35] Restivo DA, Hamdy S. Pharyngeal electrical stimulation device for the treatment of neurogenic dysphagia: Technology update. Medical Devices (Auckland). 2018;**11**:21-26. DOI: 10.2147/MDER.S122287

[36] Grandidge L, Chotiyarnwong C, White S, Denning J, Nair KPS. Survival following the placement of gastrostomy tube in patients with multiple sclerosis. Multiple Sclerosis Journal—Experimental, Translational Clinical. 2020;**6**(1):2055217319900907. DOI: 10.1177/2055217319900907

[37] Cosentino G, Gargano R, Bonura G, et al. Anodal tDCS of the swallowing motor cortex for treatment of dysphagia in multiple sclerosis: A pilot open-label study. Neurological Sciences. 2018;**39**(8):1471-1473. DOI: 10.1007/s10072-018-3443-x

[38] Restivo DA, Alfonsi E, Casabona A, et al. A pilot study on the efficacy of transcranial direct current stimulation applied to the pharyngeal motor cortex for dysphagia associated with brainstem involvement in multiple sclerosis. Clinical Neurophysiology. 2019;**130**(6):1017-1024. DOI: 10.1016/j.clinph.2019.04.003

[39] Sadeghi Z, Ghoreishi ZS, Flowers H, Mohammadkhani P, Ashtari F, Noroozi M. Depression, anxiety, and stress relative to swallowing impairment in persons with multiple sclerosis. Dysphagia. 2021;**36**(5):902-909. DOI: 10.1007/s00455-020-10207-x

[40] Cousins O, Girelli E, Harikrishnan S. Neuromyelitis optica: an elusive cause of dysphagia. BMJ Case Rep. 14 Jan 2019;**12**(1):227041. DOI: 10.1136/bcr-2018-227041

[41] Salahudeen A, Mistry T. Gastroparesis as the sole presenting feature of neuromyelitis optica. ACG Case Reports Journal. 2017;**4**:e109. DOI: 10.14309/crj.2017.109

[42] Wang Y, Zhang L, Zhang B, et al. Comparative clinical characteristics of neuromyelitis optica spectrum disorders with and without medulla oblongata lesions. Journal of Neurology. 2014;**261**(5):954-962. DOI: 10.1007/s00415-014-7298-7

[43] Pawlitzki M, Ahring S, Rolfes L, et al. Dysphagia in neuromyelitis optica spectrum disorder and myelin oligodendrocyte glycoprotein antibody disease as a surrogate of brain involvement? European Journal of Neurology. 2021;**28**(5):1765-1770. DOI: 10.1111/ene.14691

[44] Turkoglu R, Kiyat-Atamer A, Tuzun E, Akman-Demir G. Isolated dysphagia due to aquaporin-4 autoimmunity. The Turkish Journal of Gastroenterology. 2012;**23**(6):804-805. DOI: 10.4318/tjg.2012.0437

[45] Lebar R, Baudrimont M, Vincent C. Chronic experimental autoimmune encephalomyelitis in the guinea pig. Presence of anti-M2 antibodies in central nervous system tissue and the possible role of M2 autoantigen in the induction of the disease. Journal of Autoimmunity. 1989;**2**(2):115-132. DOI: 10.1016/0896-8411(89)90149-2

[46] O'Connor KC, McLaughlin KA, De Jager PL, et al. Self-antigen tetramers discriminate between myelin autoantibodies to native or denatured protein. Nature Medicine. 2007;**13**(2): 211-217. DOI: 10.1038/nm1488

[47] Armangue T, Capobianco M, de Chalus A, Laetitia G, Deiva K, Consortium EUpM. E.U. paediatric MOG consortium consensus: Part 3—Biomarkers of paediatric myelin oligodendrocyte glycoprotein antibody-associated disorders. European Journal of Paediatric Neurology. 2020;**29**:22-31. DOI: 10.1016/j.ejpn.2020.11.001

[48] Reindl M, Waters P. Myelin oligodendrocyte glycoprotein antibodies in neurological disease. Nature Reviews. Neurology. 2019;**15**(2):89-102. DOI: 10.1038/s41582-018-0112-x

[49] Jarius S, Kleiter I, Ruprecht K, et al. MOG-IgG in NMO and related disorders: A multicenter study of 50 patients. Part 3: Brainstem involvement—Frequency, presentation and outcome. Journal of Neuroinflammation. 2016;**13**(1):281. DOI: 10.1186/s12974-016-0719-z

[50] Graus F, Titulaer MJ, Balu R, et al. A clinical approach to diagnosis of autoimmune encephalitis. Lancet Neurology. 2016;**15**(4):391-404. DOI: 10.1016/S1474-4422(15)00401-9

[51] Gaig C, Graus F, Compta Y, et al. Clinical manifestations of the anti-IgLON5 disease. Neurology. 2017;**88**(18):1736-1743. DOI: 10.1212/WNL.0000000000003887

[52] Honorat JA, Komorowski L, Josephs KA, et al. IgLON5 antibody: Neurological accompaniments and outcomes in 20 patients. Neurology Neuroimmunology & Neuro inflammation. 2017;**4**(5):e385. DOI: 10.1212/NXI.0000000000000385

[53] Tobin WO, Lennon VA, Komorowski L, et al. DPPX potassium channel antibody: Frequency, clinical accompaniments, and outcomes in 20 patients. Neurology. 2014;**83**(20):1797-1803. DOI: 10.1212/WNL.000000 0000000991

[54] Castle J, Sakonju A, Dalmau J, Newman-Toker DE. Anti-Ma2-associated encephalitis with normal FDG-PET: A case of pseudo-Whipple's disease. Nature Clinical Practice. Neurology. 2006;**2**(10):566-572, quiz 573. DOI: 10.1038/ncpneuro0287

[55] Oz Tuncer G, Teber S, Kutluk MG, Albayrak P, Deda G. Hashimoto's encephalopathy presenting as pseudobulbar palsy. Child's Nervous System. 2018;**34**(6):1251-1254. DOI: 10.1007/s00381-018-3720-2

[56] Pittock SJ, Lucchinetti CF, Lennon VA. Anti-neuronal nuclear autoantibody type 2: Paraneoplastic accompaniments. Annals of Neurology. 2003;**53**(5):580-587. DOI: 10.1002/ana.10518

[57] Li XL, Han J, Zhao HT, Long YM, Zhang BW, Wang HY. Autoimmune glial fibrillary acidic protein astrocytopathy with lesions distributed predominantly in the entire spinal cord. Therapeutic Advances in Neurological Disorders. 2020;**13**:1756286420909973. DOI: 10.1177/1756286420909973

[58] Shelly S, Kryzer TJ, Komorowski L, Miske R, Anderson MD, Flanagan EP, et al. Neurochondrin neurological autoimmunity. Neurology - Neuroimmunology Neuroinflammation. 2019;**6**(6):e612. DOI: 10.1212/NXI.0000000000000612

[59] Wallwitz U, Brock S, Schunck A, Wildemann B, Jarius S, Hoffmann F. From dizziness to severe ataxia and dysarthria: New cases of anti-Ca/ARHGAP26 autoantibody-associated cerebellar ataxia suggest a broad clinical spectrum. Journal of Neuroimmunology. 15 2017;**309**:77-81. DOI: 10.1016/j.jneuroim.2017.05.011

[60] Michev A, Musso P, Foiadelli T, et al. Bickerstaff brainstem encephalitis and overlapping Guillain-Barre syndrome in children: Report of two cases and review of the literature. European Journal of Paediatric Neurology. 2019;**23**(1):43-52. DOI: 10.1016/j.ejpn.2018.11.008

[61] Dietrich-Burns K, Lewis WJ, Lesley DY, Solomon NP. Silent aspiration and recovery from dysphagia in a case of bickerstaff brainstem encephalitis. Military Medicine. 2013;**178**(1):e121-e124. DOI: 10.7205/MILMED-D-12-00268

[62] Pittard A, Abramo TJ, Arnold DH. A child with difficulty swallowing. Pediatric Emergency Care. 2009;**25**(8):525-528. DOI: 10.1097/PEC.0b013e3181b0a443

[63] Ma Y, Sun X, Li W, et al. Chronic lymphocytic inflammation with pontine perivascular enhancement responsive to steroids (CLIPPERS) with intracranial Epstein-Barr virus infection: A case report. Medicine (Baltimore). 2016;**95**(46):e5377. DOI: 10.1097/MD.0000000000005377

[64] Arma S, Habibulla KS, Price JJ, Collis JL. Dysphagia in Behcet's syndrome. Thorax. 1971;**26**(2):155-158. DOI: 10.1136/thx.26.2.155

[65] Borhani-Haghighi A, Kardeh B, Banerjee S, et al. Neuro-Behcet's disease: An update on diagnosis, differential diagnoses, and treatment. Multiple Sclerosis and Related Disorders. 2019;**39**:101906. DOI: 10.1016/j.msard.2019.101906

[66] Manasson J, Howard J, Nowatzky J. Brainstem astrocytoma as a neuro-Behçet's disease mimic. BMJ Case Rep. 7 Dec 2018;**11**(1):e226945. DOI: 10.1136/bcr-2018-226945

[67] Preziosa P, Rocca MA, Ramirez GA, et al. Structural and functional brain connectomes in patients with systemic lupus erythematosus. European Journal of Neurology. 2020;**27**(1):113-1e2. DOI: 10.1111/ene.14041

[68] Sarbu N, Alobeidi F, Toledano P, et al. Brain abnormalities in newly diagnosed neuropsychiatric lupus: Systematic MRI approach and correlation with clinical and laboratory data in a large multicenter cohort. Autoimmunity Reviews. 2015;**14**(2):153-159. DOI: 10.1016/j.autrev.2014.11.001

[69] Ebert EC, Hagspiel KD. Gastrointestinal and hepatic manifestations of systemic lupus erythematosus. Journal of Clinical Gastroenterology. 2011;**45**(5):436-441. DOI: 10.1097/MCG.0b013e31820f81b8

[70] Margaretten M. Neurologic manifestations of primary Sjogren syndrome. Rheumatic Diseases Clinics of North America. 2017;**43**(4):519-529. DOI: 10.1016/j.rdc.2017.06.002

[71] Akaishi T, Takahashi T, Fujihara K, et al. Impact of comorbid Sjogren syndrome in anti-aquaporin-4 antibody-positive neuromyelitis optica spectrum disorders. Journal of Neurology. 2021;**268**(5):1938-1944. DOI: 10.1007/s00415-020-10377-6

[72] Vivino FB, Bunya VY, Massaro-Giordano G, et al. Sjogren's syndrome: An update on disease pathogenesis, clinical manifestations and treatment. Clinical Immunology. 2019;**203**:81-121. DOI: 10.1016/j.clim.2019.04.009

[73] Ibitoye RT, Wilkins A, Scolding NJ. Neurosarcoidosis: A clinical approach to diagnosis and management. Journal of Neurology. 2017;**264**(5):1023-1028. DOI: 10.1007/s00415-016-8336-4

[74] Abdallah T, Abdallah M, Elsayegh D, et al. Isolated dysphagia unmasking bulbar neurosarcoidosis and pulmonary sarcoidosis. Arab Journal of Gastroenterology. 2014;**15**(2):85-87. DOI: 10.1016/j.ajg.2014.03.001

[75] Chaudhry HS, Ata F, Abdelghani M, Kazman R, Rahil A. Isolated Bulbar palsy: A rare presentation of neurosarcoidosis. Cureus. 2020;**12**(2): e7010. DOI: 10.7759/cureus.7010

Section 3

Dysphagia Following Surgery

Chapter 4

Dysphagia Following Anterior Cervical Spine Surgery

Ghazwan Hasan and Oscar L. Alves

Abstract

Dysphasia is regarded as one of the common complications following anterior cervical discectomy and fusion, the reported incidence varies widely and is depending on several factors, such as smoking, multi levels, anterior plating, we will discuss historical review, pathogenesis, epidemiology, clinical presentation including presentation including perioperative and postoperative recommendation and will end up with different stops and tricks to decrease this complication, in each topics we will review the evidence based articles.

Keywords: dysphagia, ACDF, cervical plating anterior cervical spine surgery

1. Introduction

Surgical approaches to the cervical spine include anterior, posterior, trans-oral, lateral trans-mandibular which can be done by open, tubular MIS or full endoscopic as described recently.

Anterior cervical spine surgery is commonly performed for the treatment of varieties of cervical spine pathologies that include degenerative, trauma, tumors, deformities and infections [1].

Techniques of anterior cervical spine surgery include anterior cervical discectomy and fusion (ACDF), anterior cervical corpectomy and fusion (ACCF), for primary stability and fusion different type of devices are used, such as cages, plates, cylinders, as well as bone growth promoters, substitutes, and bone morphogenic protein (BMP) have been use. In selected cases, discectomy alone is also performed especially through MIS or endoscopic techniques [2].

Anterior cervical discectomy and fusion (ACDF) was first described by Smith Robinson in 1968, when he performed discectomy and fusion was done using tri-cortical bone graft, during 1990s more than 500,000 anterior cervical discectomy and fusion (ACDF) was done in USA [3].

Anterior cervical spine surgery is safe and effective harboring a wide range of indications with a low rate of morbidity and mortality [4]. Complications following anterior cervical spine surgery include airway complications, dysphagia, dysphonia, infection, implant failure, non-union, neurological deficit, vascular injuries, implant subsidence, adjacent level disease and even death [5–10].

Dysphagia is one of the most common complications following anterior cervical spine surgeries, dysphagia is a symptom indicative of an abnormality in the neural control of, or the structures involved in, any phase of the swallowing process, which involve both voluntary and involuntary/reflex responses. Oropharyngeal dysphagia is an impairment in the speed and/or safe delivery of food materials from entry in the mouth to the upper portion of the esophagus. If present, the patient is at an increased risk of aspiration and may be unable to swallow properly liquids, foods, or saliva. The condition is considered long standing if it is still present more than 4 weeks after surgery [11].

Dysphagia following anterior cervical surgery can occur in the three phases of swallowing process (oral & transport phase, pharyngeal & esophageal) [12].

2. Incidence and prevalence

Postoperative dysphagia is the most common complications following ACSS, the incidence ranges between 1 and 79% [1, 11, 13]. The criteria used to define and detected dysphagia may influence the reported incidence, many factors impact the exact incidence which include:

- The severity of dysphagia (mild, moderate, or severe), most of the cases fortunately presents with mild dysphagia.

- Timing of postoperative detection (immediate postoperative <2 weeks, 2 weeks, 4–6 weeks, 8–12 weeks). The earlier the detection the higher the incidence [14, 15].

- Measurement tools (repeated questionnaires or patients self-reported). The repeated questioning provides a higher incidence than self-reported [16–18].

- Surgical Techniques & Approaches (Revision, ACSS, PCSS, Standalone cage, Cervical Plate, ACDF, ACCD, & Single vs. multilevel) Revision, ACSS, multilevel surgery, cervical plating, ACCD are associated with a higher incidence [19].

- Type and design of the study & sample size (retrospective or prospective, no. of the patients in the study, and the presence of control group or not). most of the studies are no controlled retrospective in nature with an intrinsic inability to detect preoperative swallowing difficulties, with no control group [20], the higher sample size the less incidence [21].

The incidence ranges between 28 and 57% in the intermediate and long term postoperative period (1–6 weeks), [17, 22], Riley et al. on a multicentric study that enrolled 454 patient who underwent ACSS in a multicentric study between 1998 and 2001 found that the incidence of postoperative dysphagia was 28.2, 6.8 and 7.8% at 3, 6, and 24 months, respectively, and at both 6 and 24 months the prevalence rate of persistent dysphagia was 21% [21]. On another study, the average incidence varied along the post-operative time after ACSS: 53.2% at 1 month, 31.6% at 2–4 months, 19.8% at 6 months, 16.8% at 12 months and 12.9 at 24 months [11].

Lee et al. reported an overall prevalence rate of postoperative dysphagia over time as the following: 54.0% at 1 month; 33.6% at 2 months; 18.6% at 6 months; 15.2% at 1 year; and 13.6% at 2 years [19].

Later, Riley et al. in a systematic review found that the incidence of postoperative dysphagia decreased with time after surgery and reach plateau at rate of 13–21% at one year [1].

3. Natural history

Most cases of postoperative dysphagia are mild and transient, resolving gradually within 3 months [19, 23, 24] without any specific treatment. Most of the cases of postoperative dysphagia resolve within 1 year, however, about 5–7% of cases of dysphagia after ACSS are still present 6–24 months after surgery [11].

Yue et al. reported 15% rate of dysphagia after 5 years of ACSS [24]. The predominant cause of persistent postoperative dysphagia appears to be an increase of the thickness of posterior pharyngeal wall above the upper esophageal sphincter [25].

4. Pathophysiology

Anterior cervical spine surgery impact both physiological and anatomical function of the swallowing, and these factors impact the neural, muscular & mucosal structures [19, 26]. However, in some cases dysphagia can occur in the absence of any noticed postoperative complication in anterior cervical spine surgery (ACSS).

We can summarize the etiology of dysphagia following anterior cervical spine surgery as the following:

Categories of causes	Representative conditions
Collagen diseases	Scleroderma, dermatomyositis
Conditions that give rise to fixed mechanical obstruction	Previous surgical treatment, tumor, cervical rings or webs, radiation/ radiotherapy (pharyngeal phase)
Congenital neurologic/structural disorders/malformations	Dysautonomia, cleft palate, cerebral palsy, muscular dystrophy
Iatrogenic	Medications (chemotherapy, neuroleptics, etc.); pill injury (intentional; oral preparatory phase)
Infectious	Botulism, diphtheria, Lyme disease, mucositis (herpetic lesions, cytomegalovirus, Candida, aphthous ulcers); syphilis (oral preparatory phase)
Intrinsic functional disturbances	Cricopharyngeal achalasia, Zenker diverticulum (pharyngeal phase)
Medical	Advanced chronic obstructive pulmonary disease, deconditioning, intubation (prolonged endotracheal), rheumatoid arthritis, some viral infections
Metabolic	Amyloidosis, Cushing syndrome, thyrotoxicosis, Wilson disease
Myopathic	Connective tissue disease (overlap syndrome), myotonic dystrophy, paraneoplastic syndromes, polymyositis, sarcoidosis
Neurologic	Dementia, Guillain-Barré syndrome, Huntington disease, metabolic encephalopathies, polio, postpolio syndrome, traumatic brain injury, seizure disorders, tardive dyskinesia, brainstem tumor, cerebral vascular accident
Neuromyogenic	Myopathies (inflammatory, metabolic), parkinsonism, head trauma, stroke (oral preparatory phase and pharyngeal phase)
Progressive neurologic disorders	Dystonia, progressive supranuclear palsy, oculopharyngeal dystrophy, myasthenia gravis, amyotrophic lateral sclerosis, multiple sclerosis, Parkinson's disease (oral preparatory phase and pharyngeal phase)
Neurosurgical procedures	Aneurysm clippings, anterior cervical spine surgery; resection of tumor
Structural	Extrinsic compression, cervical osteophytes, scar tissue (oral/ pharyngeal), stenosis (postsurgical/radiation/idiopathic), cricopharyngeal bar, skeletal abnormalities (pharyngeal phase)

Table 1.
Causes of oropharyngeal dysphagia according to categories, with corresponding representative conditions [11].

Approach/technique	Possible resulting condition
Operative approach (anterior)	
Dissection or retraction	Damage of the aerodigestive pathway; muscle and serosa injuries and edema; tissue damage with subsequent edema; bruising or laceration of tissues
	SLN injury, most at risk with surgery involving C3-C4 , which can cause laryngeal sensory impairment
	Injuries to the pharyngeal plexus or vagus nerve, glossopharyngeal nerve, or hypoglossal nerve (most at risk with surgery at or above C3)
	Dysfunction of the pharyngeal plexus, which affects the motility of the visceral wall
Dissection or retraction of the longus colli muscle	Muscle and subperiosteal bleeding; prevertebral soft tissue swelling
Retraction	Denervation of the pharyngeal plexus (involving the glossopharyngeal nerve and the pharyngeal branch of the vagus nerve)
Excessive or prolonged retraction	Dysphagia
	Esophageal edema, impingement, ischemia, denervation, re-perfusion injury
	Posterior pharyngeal wall edema, preventing a full epiglottic deflection
	Soft tissue fibrosis; soft tissue swelling; scar tissue formation
Significant tension during lateralization of the larynx (RLN most at risk with surgery involving C3–C4 and C5–T1)	RLN injury, which can cause vocal fold paresis or paralysis
RLN stretch injury and/or RLN compression injury from ET cuff compression	RLN palsy, which can cause vocal fold paresis or paralysis
Use of rh-BMP-2	Early local inflammatory response to rh-BMP-2 (dose-related)
Concurrent intraoperative traction on both the RLN and pharyngeal plexus	RLN injury
Other aspects of operative approach	
Direct esophageal injury	Impaired opening of the upper esophageal sphincter
	Localized denervation of portions of the esophagus and hypopharynx
	Pharyngeal wall ischemia
Hemostatic or coagulopathy	Hematoma formation
Operative technique	
Use of instrumentation	Any mechanical irritation or impingement against the esophagus
	Differences in postoperative cervical kyphotic-lordotic deformity
Thickness or anterior profile of anterior cervical plates and instrumentation	Irritation and inflammation
Plate on the esophagus	Mass effect
Use of graft	Craft (implant) protrusion, graft extrusion or cord compression
Improper halo or collar positioning	Cervical hyperextension

Abbreviations: ET, endotracheal; rhBMP-2, recombinant human bone morphogenetic protein-2; RLN, recurrent laryngeal nerve; SLN, superior laryngeal nerve.

Table 2.
Causes of oropharyngeal dysphagia according to operative approach and operative technique.

4.1 Prevertebral soft tissue swelling

Prevertebral soft tissue swelling is result of hemorrhage or intraoperative soft tissue trauma which leads to oedema which may cause transient dysfunction of the esophageal movement by impairing the upper esophageal sphincters. Nevertheless, Kang et al. failed to find a significant correlation between the thickness of prevertebral soft tissue and the incidence of dysphagia [27, 28].

4.2 Extrinsic esophageal compression

The presence of anterior cervical osteophyte, diffuse idiopathic skeletal hyperostosis can cause dysphagia secondary to mechanical impingement of esophagus, as well as inflammation causing adhesion and fibrosis.

In ACDF with plating, the presence of a plate can contributes to the same pathophysiology cause of dysphagia. Although the concept is not yet fully established, it has been proven that a thicker cervical plate is associated with a higher incidence of dysphagia [22].

Several studies confirmed that standalone cages are associated with less incidence of dysphagia when compared with ACDF with plating. However, this conclusion is not universally accepted [29].

4.3 Esophageal retraction

Retraction of esophagus during surgery to expose the anterior cervical spine is one of the possible cause of postoperative dysphagia while some studies concluded that esophageal retraction may cause ischemia of the esophageal wall which in turn compromise the motility [12], one study failed to confirm the association between the intraoperative pressure of esophageal retraction and postoperative dysphagia [30].

4.4 Neural traction

Intraoperative nerve traction or injury is another possible cause of postoperative dysphagia. Different nerves traction will cause different esophageal segment dysphagia. For example damage or traction to Hypoglossal nerve will impact the oral phase of swallowing, while injury or traction to the connection between the pharyngeal plexus and pharyngeal muscle will impact the pharyngeal phase of swallowing. Injury of the recurrent laryngeal nerve (RLN) and superior laryngeal nerve (SLN) are both operative in the development of postoperative dysphagia, reason why a sound knowledge of their anatomy and meticulous surgical technique are essential to decrease the postoperative dysphagia [11].

Anderson et al. [11] summarized the causes of oropharyngeal dysphagia as seen in **Table 1**.

Regarding the surgical techniques, the causes of dysphagia are described in **Table 2**.

5. Risk factors

5.1 Patient-related

5.1.1 Age

Smith-Hammond et al. [20] found that older patients have an higher risk of dysphagia following ACDF, while Lee et al. [19] and Bazaz et al. [19] found the no correlation between the age and the risk of dysphagia.

5.1.2 Sex

Female gender harbors an increased risk of dysphagia following ACDF [13, 19], while other studies failed to find the association between sex and dysphagia [21, 31].

5.1.3 Smoking

Many studies found that smoking is associated with and increased the risk of dysphagia following ACDF, due to its detrimental effect on soft tissue, as well as poor surgical outcomes after ACSS [5, 32].

5.1.4 Co-morbidities

Specifically the Chronic Obstructive Pulmonary Disease (COPD) increase the risk of overall postoperative mortality and morbidities following anterior cervical spine surgery [33], many studies were found the risk of dysphagia is increase in patients with COPD following ACDF [32].

5.2 Surgery-related

5.2.1 Duration of surgery

The longer the surgical time, which happens in complex procedures or in surgeries performed by less experienced surgeons, the higher contribution to the development of dysphagia, although some studies failed conclude it.

5.2.2 Multilevel surgery

Some studies have shown that multiple levels surgeries represent a significant risk factor for dysphagia [19], however others did not find any correlation between the multilevel and risk of dysphagia [31].

5.2.3 Revision surgery

In cases of revision surgeries, the presence of scar tissue can distort the anatomy compared to index surgery, rendering esophageal injury more likely [19].

5.2.4 Implant

Depending on the surgical indications related to the pathology, the level affected and the presence of deformity, different implants are used in anterior cervical surgeries. According to his/her experience and preferences, the surgeon may use stand-alone cage, hybrid cage, cervical plating, or total disc replacement [34].

The use of cervical plate in ACDF remain a controversy issue, especially in single and two levels degenerative disc disease, but many studies support its use in more than 2 levels in degenerative spine, in trauma, tumor, infections, especially if corpectomies are advocated.

Plating has the advantage of increase fusion rate, better lordotic reconstruction, enhanced primary stability of the construct, superior disc height preservation and lower subsidence rate [35]. However these benefits come at the cost of screw pullout, loosening of plate, hardware breakage, increase in the operative time and overall costs, and increased risk of dysphagia [34].

Total disc arthroplasty (TDR) become popularized in last decades as a motion preserving technique in the anterior cervical surgeries, avoiding the fusion and decrease the adverse effect of ACDF, in selected indications. However, studies found no difference in the risk of dysphagia when comparing between TDR and ACDF [36].

5.2.5 Bone morphogenetic protein (BMP)

Bone morphogenetic protein is used during cervical surgery to increase the fusion rate especially in cases of accrued risk of pseudoarthrosis. Some studies found that BMP may constitute a risk factor for dysphagia following ACDF as it induces inflammation and oedema which will affect the surrounding soft tissue, including the esophagus [37, 38].

5.2.6 Surgical level: several

Studies found that a high level of cervical spine surgery, such as C3-4, is associated with more dysphagia than the lower levels. In the upper cervical spine, the risk of superior laryngeal nerve injury is amplified which entails an increased risk of dysphagia. As the retropharyngeal space in the upper cervical spine is more generous than in inferior cervical spine, the soft tissue swelling will be potentially more severe [39].

5.2.7 Blood loss

Significant blood loss impacts in the overall surgical outcome and is associated with many adverse effects that includes postoperative recovery and infection rate. In fact, some studies have shown than blood loss superior to 300 ml is associated with an enhanced risk of dysphagia following ACSS [21].

6. Clinical signs and symptoms

Patients present with dysphagia due to alteration in swallowing mechanisms that include [25]:

- Increased aspiration.
- Thickening of the pharyngeal wall.
- Poorer pharyngeal constriction and peristalsis.
- Prolonged transit time.
- Reduced hyoid displacement.
- Reduced opening of the pharyngoesophageal segment opening.
- Impaired epiglottic inversion

As a result of dysphagia, patients may develop other symptoms that may include:

- Reflexive coughing or wet/gurgle voice during or right after swallowing.
- Extra effort or time needed to chew or swallow.
- Food or liquid leaking from the mouth or getting stuck in the mouth.
- Recurring pneumonia or chest congestion after eating.

Persistent & severe dysphagia may result in weight loss, dehydration, risk of aspiration pneumonia, chronic lung disease and psychological problems [40].

The presence of long-standing dysphagia should raise the suspicion of esophageal perforation and thus be adamantly investigated.

7. Assessment and evaluation

7.1 Patient-reported outcome

Non-validated questionaries to evaluate the severity of dysphagia following ACSS include:

7.1.1 Bazaz dysphagia questionnaire

Depending on liquid and/or solid food difficulty swelling, they graded the severity into none, mild, moderate, and severe, as described in **Table 3** [13].

7.1.2 Modified Bazaz questionnaire

It is a modification of Bazaz Dysphagia Score into a ten-points scale recorded daily for four days, with dysphagia being defined as a cumulative four-day score of ≥12 [30]. As seen in **Table 4**.

Severity of dysphagia	Difficulty swallowing liquids	Difficulty swallowing solids
None	None	None
Mild	None	Rare
Moderate	None or rare	Occasionally (only with specific foods)
Severe	None or rare	Frequent (majority of solids)

Table 3.
Bazaz dysphagia scoring system [2].

Points	Severity of dysphagia	Definition
0	None	No episodes of difficulty swallowing
1–3	Mild	Only rare episodes of difficulty swallowing
4–6	Moderate	Occasional swallowing difficulty with solid foods
7–10	Severe	Swallowing difficulty with solids and liquids

Table 4.
Modified Bazaz dysphagia scoring system [15]. Assessment is undertaken on the day of operation and on the first, third and fifth post-operative days; the scores are added together, with dysphagia defined as a cumulative score of ≥ 12.

7.1.3 Dysphagia numerical rating scale

Assess the postoperative dysphagia using numeric scale [31].

7.1.4 Dysphagia disability index

Includes also physical function and emotional domains [31].

7.1.5 Swallowing-quality of life (SWAL-QOL) questionnaire

Swallowing-quality of life (SWAL-QOL) questionnaire is a validated 93-item questionnaire that quantifies dysphagia on the basis of severity and duration as well as its psychological impact [32], although it is has been shown to be valid and reliable, its length and complexity make it less practical in the clinical setting.

7.2 Videoflouroscopic swallow evaluation (VSE)

Videoflouroscopic swallow evaluation (VSE) is a gold standard for the assessment of swallowing impairment also referred to as a modified barium swallow study [41].

8. Treatment

The aim of treatment in postoperative dysphagia following ACSS is to maximize the food transit, minimize or prevent respiratory aspiration and related adverse effect [42].

Currently there is no specific treatment for dysphagia, as many patients with postoperative dysphagia will resolve with time. The available treatment include behavioral, postural changes, sensory input enhancement, swallowing maneuvers, voluntary control in effort exerted during swallowing and diet modification [43].

The best form of treatment is prevention, as discussed in the next section.

For persistent dysphagia that extends for more than 12–18 months, some authors recommend surgical treatment to debride the adhesion or anterior cervical instrumentation to immobilize the spine to avoid esophagus tethering and traction [44].

9. Prevention

Many studies evaluated the techniques and recommendation to decrease the incidence of postoperative dysphasia following ACSS.

9.1 Steroid therapy

The intra-operative local application of steroids in is regarded as a preventive measure to abort the development of postoperative dysphagia. This is based on the pathogenesis, as soft tissue swelling, and local inflammation will be decrease when the steroids are used. In this respect the use of IV Methylprednisolone is recommended [45], while the local application of triamcinolone in the retropharyngeal space may decrease the incidence of dysphagia postoperatively [46].

9.2 Endotracheal tube pressure

Excessive endotracheal tube pressure may impact locally by increasing transmural pressure translating in a putative risk of soft tissue injury and dysphagia development following ACSS, Accordingly, some authors recommend decreasing the endotracheal tube pressure to 20 mmHg during the period of cervical traction [47], or the release of the endotracheal tube pressure and reinflate it after retractor placement to minimize the pressure related damage to the RLN [48].

9.3 Cervical plate design

A plate can cause postoperative dysphagia due to mass effect or induction of inflammation, plate redesign to a low profile by decreasing its thickness will endure a minimization of postoperative dysphagia [22]. Equally, the use of a zero profile cage and plate or hybrid cage has shown a smaller incidence of postoperative dysphagia [49].

9.4 Tracheal traction exercises

The concept behind the preoperative tracheal traction exercise is to increase the compliance of the esophagus, thereby reducing the pressure required by retraction to expose an adequate operative field, the exercises were performed twice daily (15 times each time) for three days, starting four days before the operation [50].

9.5 Surgical techniques

An effort to limit the operative time should be undertaken to decrease the postoperative dysphagia. Appropriate surgical training should focus on acquiring a sound knowledge of anatomical variation of the RLN & SLN, a meticulous plan by plan surgical dissection, control of blood loss to better identify anatomical structures, avoid excessive blade retraction to reduce mechanical transmural esophageal pressure and anchoring the blades under the dissected longus coli to avoid injury to RLN and SLN [11, 48, 51].

10. Conclusion

Dysphagia following anterior cervical spine surgery is a common complication, in most cases it is mild and resolved with time, no specific treatment is required.

There are risk factors to increase the risk that include multiple levels, smoking, cervical plating, increase the operative time, revision surgeries.

Conflict of interest

The authors declare no conflict of interest.

Author details

Ghazwan Hasan[1*] and Oscar L. Alves[2]

1 Royal Private Hospital, Baghdad, Iraq

2 Department of Neurosurgery, Centro Hospitalar de Vila Nova de Gaia, Porto, Portugal

*Address all correspondence to: dr.bayaty@gmail.com

References

[1] Riley LH 3rd, Vaccaro AR, Dettori JR, Hashimoto R. Postoperative dysphagia in anterior cervical spine surgery. Spine (Phila Pa 1976). 2010;**35**(Suppl. 9): S76-S85

[2] Quillo-Olvera J, Lin GX, Kim JS. Percutaneous endoscopic cervical discectomy: A technical review. Annals of Translational Medicine. 2018; **6**(6):100

[3] Angevine PD, Arons RR, McCormick PC. National and regional rates and variation of cervical discectomy with and without anterior fusion, 1990-1999. Spine (Phila Pa 1976). 2003;**28**(9):931-939; discussion 40

[4] Wang H, Meng Y, Liu H, Wang X, Hong Y. The impact of smoking on outcomes following anterior cervical fusion-nonfusion hybrid surgery: A retrospective single-center cohort study. BMC Musculoskeletal Disorders. 2021;**22**(1):612

[5] Hasan GARH, Al-Naser LM, Sheta RA. Early complications of anterior cervical discectomy and fusion: A case series. Journal of Musculoskeletal Surgery and Research. 2018;**2**:121-125

[6] Fountas KN, Kapsalaki EZ, Nikolakakos LG, Smisson HF, Johnston KW, Grigorian AA, et al. Anterior cervical discectomy and fusion associated complications. Spine (Phila Pa 1976). 2007;**32**(21):2310-2317

[7] Cheung ZB, Gidumal S, White S, Shin J, Phan K, Osman N, et al. Comparison of anterior cervical discectomy and fusion with a stand-alone interbody cage versus a conventional cage-plate technique: A systematic review and meta-analysis. Global Spine Journal. 2019;**9**(4): 446-455

[8] Kashkoush A, Mehta A, Agarwal N, Nwachuku EL, Fields DP, Alan N, et al. Perioperative neurological complications following anterior cervical discectomy and fusion: Clinical impact on 317,789 patients from the national inpatient sample. World Neurosurgery. 2019;**128**:e107-ee15

[9] Wewel JT, Kasliwal MK, Adogwa O, Deutsch H, O'Toole JE, Traynelis VC. Fusion rate following three- and four-level ACDF using allograft and segmental instrumentation: A radiographic study. Journal of Clinical Neuroscience. 2019;**62**:142-146

[10] Narain AS, Hijji FY, Haws BE, Khechen B, Kudaravalli KT, Yom KH, et al. Risk factors for medical and surgical complications after 1-2-level anterior cervical discectomy and fusion procedures. International Journal of Spine Surgery. 2020;**14**(3):286-293

[11] Anderson KK, Arnold PM. Oropharyngeal dysphagia after anterior cervical spine surgery: A review. Global Spine Journal. 2013;**3**(4):273-286

[12] Mendoza-Lattes S, Clifford K, Bartelt R, Stewart J, Clark CR, Boezaart AP. Dysphagia following anterior cervical arthrodesis is associated with continuous, strong retraction of the esophagus. The Journal of Bone and Joint Surgery. American Volume. 2008;**90**(2):256-263

[13] Bazaz R, Lee MJ, Yoo JU. Incidence of dysphagia after anterior cervical spine surgery: A prospective study. Spine (Phila Pa 1976). 2002;**27**(22): 2453-2458

[14] Tervonen H, Niemelä M, Lauri ER, Back L, Juvas A, Räsänen P, et al. Dysphonia and dysphagia after anterior cervical decompression. Journal of Neurosurgery. Spine. 2007;**7**(2):124-130

[15] Vaidya R, Carp J, Sethi A, Bartol S, Craig J, Les CM. Complications of anterior cervical discectomy and fusion using recombinant human bone morphogenetic protein-2. European Spine Journal. 2007;**16**(8):1257-1265

[16] Danto J, DiCapua J, Nardi D, Pekmezaris R, Moise G, Lesser M, et al. Multiple cervical levels: Increased risk of dysphagia and dysphonia during anterior cervical discectomy. Journal of Neurosurgical Anesthesiology. 2012;**24**(4):350-355

[17] Edwards CC 2nd, Karpitskaya Y, Cha C, Heller JG, Lauryssen C, Yoon ST, et al. Accurate identification of adverse outcomes after cervical spine surgery. The Journal of Bone and Joint Surgery. American Volume. 2004;**86**(2):251-256

[18] Cho SK, Lu Y, Lee DH. Dysphagia following anterior cervical spinal surgery: A systematic review. Bone & Joint Journal. 2013;**95-b**(7):868-873

[19] Lee MJ, Bazaz R, Furey CG, Yoo J. Risk factors for dysphagia after anterior cervical spine surgery: A two-year prospective cohort study. The Spine Journal. 2007;7(2):141-147

[20] Smith-Hammond CA, New KC, Pietrobon R, Curtis DJ, Scharver CH, Turner DA. Prospective analysis of incidence and risk factors of dysphagia in spine surgery patients: Comparison of anterior cervical, posterior cervical, and lumbar procedures. Spine (Phila Pa 1976). 2004;**29**(13):1441-1446

[21] Riley LH 3rd, Skolasky RL, Albert TJ, Vaccaro AR, Heller JG. Dysphagia after anterior cervical decompression and fusion: Prevalence and risk factors from a longitudinal cohort study. Spine (Phila Pa 1976). 2005;**30**(22):2564-2569

[22] Lee MJ, Bazaz R, Furey CG, Yoo J. Influence of anterior cervical plate design on Dysphagia: A 2-year prospective longitudinal follow-up study. Journal of Spinal Disorders & Techniques. 2005;**18**(5):406-409

[23] Kasimatis GB, Panagiotopoulos E, Gliatis J, Tyllianakis M, Zouboulis P, Lambiris E. Complications of anterior surgery in cervical spine trauma: An overview. Clinical Neurology and Neurosurgery. 2009;**111**(1):18-27

[24] Yue WM, Brodner W, Highland TR. Persistent swallowing and voice problems after anterior cervical discectomy and fusion with allograft and plating: A 5- to 11-year follow-up study. European Spine Journal. 2005;**14**(7):677-682

[25] Leonard R, Belafsky P. Dysphagia following cervical spine surgery with anterior instrumentation: Evidence from fluoroscopic swallow studies. Spine (Phila Pa 1976). 2011;**36**(25):2217-2223

[26] Pattavilakom A, Seex KA. Results of a prospective randomized study comparing a novel retractor with a Caspar retractor in anterior cervical surgery. Neurosurgery. 2011;**69**(2 Suppl Operative):ons156-ons160; discussion ons60

[27] Frempong-Boadu A, Houten JK, Osborn B, Opulencia J, Kells L, Guida DD, et al. Swallowing and speech dysfunction in patients undergoing anterior cervical discectomy and fusion: A prospective, objective preoperative and postoperative assessment. Journal of Spinal Disorders & Techniques. 2002;**15**(5):362-368

[28] Kang SH, Kim DK, Seo KM, Kim KT, Kim YB. Multi-level spinal fusion and postoperative prevertebral thickness increase the risk of dysphagia after anterior cervical spine surgery. Journal of Clinical Neuroscience. 2011;**18**(10):1369-1373

[29] Chin KR, Eiszner JR, Adams SB Jr. Role of plate thickness as a cause of dysphagia after anterior cervical fusion. Spine (Phila Pa 1976). 2007;**32**(23): 2585-2590

[30] Papavero L, Heese O, Klotz-Regener V, Buchalla R, Schröder F, Westphal M. The impact of esophagus retraction on early dysphagia after anterior cervical surgery: Does a correlation exist? Spine (Phila Pa 1976). 2007;**32**(10):1089-1093

[31] Rihn JA, Kane J, Albert TJ, Vaccaro AR, Hilibrand AS. What is the incidence and severity of dysphagia after anterior cervical surgery? Clinical Orthopaedics and Related Research. 2011;**469**(3):658-665

[32] Siska PA, Ponnappan RK, Hohl JB, Lee JY, Kang JD, Donaldson WF 3rd. Dysphagia after anterior cervical spine surgery: A prospective study using the swallowing-quality of life questionnaire and analysis of patient comorbidities. Spine (Phila Pa 1976). 2011;**36**(17): 1387-1391

[33] Malik AT, Jain N, Kim J, Khan SN, Yu E. Chronic obstructive pulmonary disease is an independent predictor for 30-day complications and readmissions following 1- to 2-level anterior cervical discectomy and fusion. Global Spine Journal. 2019;**9**(3):298-302

[34] Viswanathan VK, Manoharan SR. To plate or not to plate after a single- or two-level anterior cervical discectomy: Fusion with cage-plate construct or stand-alone cage. Asian Spine Journal. 2017;**11**(1):1-3

[35] Song KJ, Taghavi CE, Lee KB, Song JH, Eun JP. The efficacy of plate construct augmentation versus cage alone in anterior cervical fusion. Spine (Phila Pa 1976). 2009;**34**(26):2886-2892

[36] Anderson PA, Nassr A, Currier BL, Sebastian AS, Arnold PM, Fehlings MG, et al. Evaluation of adverse events in total disc replacement: A meta-analysis of fda summary of safety and effectiveness data. Global Spine Journal. 2017;**7**(Suppl. 1):76s-83s

[37] Buttermann GR. Prospective nonrandomized comparison of an allograft with bone morphogenic protein versus an iliac-crest autograft in anterior cervical discectomy and fusion. The Spine Journal. 2008;**8**(3):426-435

[38] Ozgursoy OB, Salassa JR, Reimer R, Wharen RE, Deen HG. Anterior cervical osteophyte dysphagia: Manofluorographic and functional outcomes after surgery. Head & Neck. 2010;**32**(5):588-593

[39] Liu F-Y, Yang D-L, Huang W-Z, Huo L-S, Ma L, Wang H, et al. Risk factors for dysphagia after anterior cervical spine surgery: A meta-analysis. Medicine. 2017;**96**(10):e6267

[40] Cook IJ, Kahrilas PJ. AGA technical review on management of oropharyngeal dysphagia. Gastroenterology. 1999;**116**(2):455-478

[41] Martin-Harris B, Brodsky MB, Michel Y, Castell DO, Schleicher M, Sandidge J, et al. MBS measurement tool for swallow impairment—MBSImp: Establishing a standard. Dysphagia. 2008;**23**(4):392-405

[42] Cook IJ. Diagnostic evaluation of dysphagia. Nature Clinical Practice. Gastroenterology & Hepatology. 2008;**5**(7):393-403

[43] Logemann JA, Larsen K. Oropharyngeal dysphagia: Pathophysiology and diagnosis for the anniversary issue of diseases of the esophagus. Diseases of the Esophagus. 2012;**25**(4):299-304

[44] Fogel GR, McDonnell MF. Surgical treatment of dysphagia after anterior cervical interbody fusion. The Spine Journal. 2005;**5**(2):140-144

[45] Pedram M, Castagnera L, Carat X, Macouillard G, Vital JM. Pharyngolaryngeal lesions in patients undergoing cervical spine surgery through the anterior approach: Contribution of methylprednisolone. European Spine Journal. 2003; **12**(1):84-90

[46] Lee SH, Kim KT, Suk KS, Park KJ, Oh KI. Effect of retropharyngeal steroid on prevertebral soft tissue swelling following anterior cervical discectomy and fusion: A prospective, randomized study. Spine (Phila Pa 1976). 2011; **36**(26):2286-2292

[47] Ratnaraj J, Todorov A, McHugh T, Cheng MA, Lauryssen C. Effects of decreasing endotracheal tube cuff pressures during neck retraction for anterior cervical spine surgery. Journal of Neurosurgery. 2002;**97**(Suppl. 2): 176-179

[48] Apfelbaum RI, Kriskovich MD, Haller JR. On the incidence, cause, and prevention of recurrent laryngeal nerve palsies during anterior cervical spine surgery. Spine (Phila Pa 1976). 2000;**25**(22):2906-2912

[49] Scholz M, Schnake KJ, Pingel A, Hoffmann R, Kandziora F. A new zero-profile implant for stand-alone anterior cervical interbody fusion. Clinical Orthopaedics and Related Research. 2011;**469**(3):666-673

[50] Chen Z, Wei X, Li F, He P, Huang X, Zhang F, et al. Tracheal traction exercise reduces the occurrence of postoperative dysphagia after anterior cervical spine surgery. Spine (Phila Pa 1976). 2012;**37**(15):1292-1296

[51] Razfar A, Sadr-Hosseini SM, Rosen CA, Snyderman CH, Gooding W, Abla AA, et al. Prevention and management of dysphonia during anterior cervical spine surgery. The Laryngoscope. 2012;**122**(10):2179-2183

Section 4

Management of Dysphagia

Chapter 5

Nutrition Management in Neurogenic Dysphagia

Marina V. Petrova, Alexandr E. Shestopalov, Alexandra V. Yakovleva, Pranil Pradhan and Alexey A. Yakovlev

Abstract

Neurogenic dysphagia is an increasingly common problem. This chapter describes current approaches to enteral nutrition in patients with neurogenic dysphagia. We have shown the possibilities and our experience of using diet with a measured degree of density, specialized thickeners for drinks and food, ready-made enteral mixtures. We also identified patients who need a nasogastric tube or gastrostomy.

Keywords: neurogenic dysphagia, diet, nasogastric tube, gastrostomy tube, thickeners, dense enteral feeding mixtures

1. Introduction

The term "dysphagia" means difficulty in swallowing that a person experiences either during the primary phases of swallowing (usually described as" oropharyngeal dysphagia") or when solid food or liquid is blocked or even passed through with difficulty during its passage from the mouth to the stomach (usually described as "esophageal dysphagia"). Thus, dysphagia is a feeling of an obstacle to the typical passage of ingested food.

The problem of dysphagia of various origins is widespread. The 2011 study in the United Kingdom shows a prevalence of dysphagia in 11% of the general population [1, 2]. Dysphagia develops in 40–70% of stroke patients, 60–80% of patients with neurodegenerative diseases, in almost 13% of adults aged over 65 years, and in more than 51% of elderly patients in nursing homes [3–6]. From a study in Russia, the incidence of dysphagia in hospitals reaches up to 33% and up to 30–40% at home care [5, 7]. Dysphagia is often a prominent condition in various neurological diseases.

The risk of this pathology lies in the high probability of developing formidable complications—malnutrition, dehydration, weight loss, airway obstruction, aspiration pneumonia. Malnutrition with dysphagia is detected during the first week after a stroke in 48.3% of cases, without dysphagia in 13.6% (several authors stated that this complication occurs in 75% of cases). Malnutrition resulting from dysphagia complicates the course of the underlying disease due to the activation of catabolic processes. Among patients requiring long-term rehabilitation, malnutrition can be as high as 50% [1, 8, 9]. Malnutrition syndrome increases susceptibility to oropharyngeal flora, increases the risk of developing septic complications, leads to suppression of the immune status, reduces the strength of the cough push, reduces the level of wakefulness, impedes the implementation of rehabilitation measures. Aspiration is one of the most severe complications of dysphagia, leading to airway obstruction, aspiration pneumonia [10–12].

Dysphagia—it is a frequent and sometimes even life-threatening complication in patients with central nervous system injury. In patients with a low level of consciousness, dysphagia can cause severe destructive pneumonia, respiratory failure, and death. Nevertheless, even with a preserved level of consciousness, the fact that the presence of dysphagia carries a potential risk of aspiration and asphyxia and this fear of aspiration makes patients with speech disorders avoid taking liquid diet, which leads to dehydration of the body, which is diagnosed by doctors quite late [13, 14].

In addition to such severe complications as aspiration, destructive pneumonia, patients with dysphagia have a high risk of developing protein-energy malnutrition (PEM) due to a reduction in substrate supply. In turn, this problem worsens the quality of life and complicates the course of infectious processes, complicates wound healing, and significantly reduces physical activity [15–19]. In combination with dysphagia (moderate and severe), protein-energy malnutrition is a significant problem in patients with pressure sores. At the same time, the risk of developing pressure ulcers increases in the presence of severe concomitant pathology (spastic paresis, diabetes mellitus, destructive pneumonia), which often accompanies patients with severe brain damage. If the patient is in a chronic critical illness (CCI), the rate of pressure ulcers can reach 80%, despite ongoing preventive measures [20–23].

There are several approaches to nutritional support for neurological patients in the clinic, depending on the severity of dysphagia.

2. Diet with a measured degree of density

The first method aimed not to change the physiology of swallowing (such as surgical or rehabilitation methods) but to improve the passage of the food bolus from the oral cavity into the esophagus and reduce the risk of aspiration. In the case of an acute illness, a diet with a modified degree of density allows starting oral nutrition earlier, reducing the risk of developing disorders in the cerebral cortex's swallowing centers, and preventing digestive disorders. With progressive neurological diseases, this diet helps maintain the natural way of eating as long as possible and improves the quality of life [4, 9, 24]. However, this method also has many disadvantages:

- labor intensity; in a hospital setting, it becomes necessary to create an additional specialized therapeutic diet, which may not consider the patient's characteristics.

- limited use; this method can be safe only in the absence of aspiration, and with progressive neurological disease, there is still a risk of micro aspiration.

Thus, a diet with a certain degree of thickening is suitable for patients with mild dysphagia. From the point of view of economic feasibility, this diet is more applicable at home and in hospitals specializing in neurogenic dysphagia. In the conditions of emergency hospitals, where there are few patients with mild dysphagia, the described method, in our opinion, is too strenuous.

3. Use of nasogastric tube or gastrostomy tube for feeding

This method is justified in severe dysphagia or the absence of sufficient fruitful contact with the patient. Of course, tube feeding is also necessary for acute illness. However, tube feeding disrupts the digestion process in the oral cavity, disrupting synchronization of the secretion of the digestive glands and the entry of the food lump into the lumen of the stomach and intestines, and significantly reduces the quality of life. Moreover, tube feeding does not improve the survival rate of patients with chronic neurological diseases (for example, with dementia) [11, 25–28].

Percutaneous endoscopic gastrostomy (PEG) has several advantages over the nasogastric tube for dysphagia, notably after strokes and severe traumatic brain injury. The gastrostomy tube is more convenient from the point of view of care, and its unconscious or spontaneous removal is less likely. Also, according to several studies, patients with PEG usually receive a sufficient amount of enteral nutrition and, accordingly, have better indicators of nutritional status in comparison with a nasogastric tube [29]. In addition, prolonged standing of the nasogastric tube has a high risk of complications (such as pressure ulcers of the nasal mucosa, esophagus), significantly limits the volume of speech therapy, and may even contribute to the progression of dysphagia. Therefore, it is essential for the timely placement of gastrostomy tubes in such patients. According to clinical guidelines, the placement of a gastrostomy is necessary no later than 4 weeks of using a nasogastric tube or earlier if it is evident that the patient will not be able to return to eating through natural routes soon [5, 7, 30]. Introducing a gastrostomy tube facilitates the work of a speech therapist, increases the effectiveness of rehabilitation measures, and can accelerate the positive dynamics of dysphagia treatment.

4. Use of specialized thickeners

The most crucial point in the treatment of dysphagia is the selection of the food consistency [30–32]. The modern functional food market now offers specialized products for enteral oral nutrition with varying degrees of thickening. Products of the *NUTRI* company are of great scientific and clinical interest in this regard. Nevertheless, in our practice, we used the *Softia S* product to solve swallowing problems (fluids) and facilitate the swallowing of solid food, the *Softia G* product, based on xanthan gum, made it possible to expand thtient's diet[1].

We have conducted a study of the effectiveness of the use of these products. The Federal State Budgetary Scientific Institution "Federal Research and Clinical Center of Intensive Care Medicine and Rehabilitology" approved the studies; protocol No. 5/19 dated December 26, 2019.

Comparison of two groups (primary—*Softia S, Softia G*; control—standard diet) numerically was carried out using the nonparametric Mann-Whitney method. We compared three or more groups in terms of quantitative variables using the nonparametric Kruskal-Wallis method. The statistical significance of the differences between groups for paired and nominal indicators was carried out using the Pearson Chi-square (χ^2) and McNeimer tests in the case of independent and dependent groups, respectively. Relationship analysis was performed using Spearman's nonparametric rank correlation. The analysis of dependent indicators in the case of comparing two periods was carried out based on the Wilcoxon nonparametric test. In the case of comparing three or more measurements, the Friedman nonparametric

[1] Instructions for use of *Softia S*. http://nutri-us.com/products/softias/index.html and instructions for use of *Softia G*. http://nutri-us.com/products/softiau/index.html [Accessed: September 14, 2021].

test is used. The level of statistical significance was fixed at 0.05. Statistical data processing was performed using Statistica 10 and SAS JMP 11 software packages.

4.1 Product Softia S

According to the initial speech therapy assessment data, all patients had a mild degree of neurogenic dysphagia. According to the instrumental assessment of swallowing function on the Rosenbek scale (PAS), four patients had an aspiration rating of 3 (food enters the airways, remains above the vocal cords, but is not excreted from the airways), 26 patients had an aspiration rating of 2 (food enters the airways, stays above the vocal cords, and clears his throat from the airways). On the Fiberoptic Endoscopic Dysphagia Severity Scale (FEDSS) scale, all patients had a penetration score of 3 (fluid penetration with an excellent protective reflex).

By the end of the study, eight people of the primary group showed restoration of the swallowing function; residual effects of choking persisted in seven people. In the control group, we observed a slight improvement in two patients. In the remaining 13, changes in the degree of dysphagia were not observed (**Table 1**). Laboratory parameters and the bodyweight of patients during the observation period in both groups did not change significantly. In addition, there were no cases of pyrexia during the observation period.

To test the hypothesis about significant changes that occurred during the periods "Day 1," "Day 3," "Day 5," "Day 7," and "Day 14," a statistical analysis was carried out. In the considered period in the category "Breakfast," four out of 16 indicator changes were statistically significant. The most significant changes were found for the indicators "Food consumption time, thickener" (on average, 3.7 min; $p = 0.0033$); "The number of chokes after fluid intake, thickener" (on average, 7.0 min; $p < 0.0001$); "Number of chokes during fluid intake, thickener" (average for 8.8 min; $p < 0.0001$). On the other hand, the minor changes between periods are observed for the following indicators: "Calorie content, control," "F" (fats), and "C" (carbohydrates) ($p > 0.6184$) (**Table 1**).

In the considered period in the "Lunch" category, three out of 16 indicators change statistically significantly. The most significant changes were found for the indicators "Number of chokes after hydration, thickener" (on average, 8.1 min; $p < 0.0001$); "The number of chokes during fluid intake, thickener" (on average, 12.1 min; $p < 0.0001$); "Food consumption time, thickener" (on average, 6.9 min; $p < 0.0001$). On the other hand, the smallest changes between periods were observed for the following indicators: "Number of chokes after fluid intake, control," "Food consumption time, control," and "C" (carbohydrates) ($p > 0.6015$) (**Table 2**).

In the considered period in the category "Dinner," eight out of 16 indicators change statistically significantly. The most significant changes were found for the indicators "Number of chokes after fluid intake, thickener" (on average, 6.8 min; $p < 0.0001$); "The number of chokes during fluid intake, thickener" (average of 8.7 min; $p < 0.0001$). On the other hand, the pettiest changes between periods were observed for the following indicators: "P" (protein), "Number of chokes after fluid intake, control," and "Amount of fluid consumed, control" ($p > 0.4098$) (**Table 3**).

Assessing qualitative indicator dynamics (the presence or absence of dysphonia with sputum), statistically significant differences in the dynamics of dysphonia from the 1st to the 14th day of the study were revealed in the primary group all meals. In contrast, in the control group, there were no significant differences (**Table 4**).

4.2 Product Softia G

The duration of the study was 28 days. For the first 14 days, patients received a standard hospital diet, then for another 14 days—a diet supplemented with Softia

DOI: http://dx.doi.org/10.5772/intechopen.101798

Groups	Index	M ± S	M ± S (%)				p
		Day 1	Day 3	Day 5	Day 7	Day 14	
Thickener	Food consumption time, min	32.93 ± 5.57	31.87 ± 5.72 (−3.24)	32.13 ± 5.88 (−2.43)	31.80 ± 5.66 (−3.44)	29.27 ± 5.73 (−11.13)	0.0033
Thickener	Number of chocks during fluid intake	9.80 ± 4.16	8.80 ± 3.78 (−10.20)	6.80 ± 3.76 (−30.61)	5.00 ± 3.68 (−48.98)	1.00 ± 1.31 (−89.80)	<0.0001
Thickener	Number of chocks after fluid intake	7.60 ± 3.64	6.60 ± 3.52 (−13.16)	5.27 ± 3.43 (−30.70)	3.93 ± 3.35 (−48.25)	0.60 ± 0.83 (−92.11)	<0.0001
Thickener	Calorie content	410.28 ± 48.14	454.82 ± 82.89 (10.85)	445.15 ± 57.42 (8.50)	421.65 ± 57.36 (2.77)	416.85 ± 63.71 (1.60)	0.4022
Thickener	P (proteins)	16.27 ± 4.32	18.62 ± 3.95 (14.44)	16.37 ± 2.40 (0.59)	17.58 ± 4.97 (8.04)	17.58 ± 4.97 (8.04)	0.0289
Thickener	F (fats)	17.95 ± 5.05	21.12 ± 3.94 (17.61)	22.43 ± 9.72 (24.90)	22.11 ± 8.03 (23.12)	22.11 ± 8.03 (23.12)	0.8652
Thickener	C (carbohydrates)	50.89 ± 21.36	46.04 ± 17.31 (−9.52)	52.53 ± 12.49 (3.23)	55.03 ± 28.42 (8.15)	48.37 ± 25.85 (−4.95)	0.2491
Thickener	Amount of fluid intake	232.00 ± 24.55	227.33 ± 23.74 (−2.01)	222.00 ± 23.36 (−4.31)	218.00 ± 23.96 (−6.03)	218.67 ± 21.34 (−5.75)	0.5255
Control	Food consumption time, min	34.20 ± 1.66	33.73 ± 1.98 (−1.36)	33.87 ± 2.50 (−0.97)	33.53 ± 2.26 (−1.95)	33.27 ± 1.22 (−2.73)	0.3533
Control	Number of chocks during fluid intake	10.60 ± 3.11	10.87 ± 2.92 (2.52)	10.13 ± 2.77 (−4.40)	10.60 ± 2.90 (0.00)	10.20 ± 3.69 (−3.77)	0.1532
Control	Number of chocks after fluid intake	8.40 ± 2.97	9.00 ± 3.00 (7.14)	8.60 ± 2.82 (2.38)	8.67 ± 2.79 (3.17)	8.20 ± 3.38 (−2.38)	0.3317
Control	Calorie content	452.83 ± 93.07	447.25 ± 85.48 (−1.23)	429.08 ± 63.31 (−5.24)	412.03 ± 62.98 (−9.01)	412.03 ± 62.98 (−9.01)	0.6184
Control	P (proteins)	19.55 ± 5.90	18.00 ± 4.81 (−7.94)	16.76 ± 3.39 (−14.28)	18.00 ± 5.34 (−7.94)	18.20 ± 5.25 (−6.91)	0.5710
Control	F (fats)	26.92 ± 9.89	19.69 ± 5.21 (−26.84)	20.55 ± 8.14 (−23.65)	25.32 ± 9.22 (−5.94)	25.32 ± 9.22 (−5.94)	0.0515
Control	C (carbohydrates)	53.11 ± 25.48	48.99 ± 18.41 (−7.75)	48.17 ± 13.04 (−9.30)	56.46 ± 32.78 (6.31)	56.46 ± 32.78 (6.31)	0.9939
Control	Amount of fluid intake	212.00 ± 15.21	210.67 ± 14.38 (−0.63)	214.67 ± 18.85 (1.26)	214.67 ± 16.42 (1.26)	208.00 ± 16.12 (−1.89)	0.2101

statistically significant differences in indicators are highlighted in color, the p level is presented between the indicators "Day 1" and "Day 14."

Table 1.
Analysis of the dynamics of quantitative indicators for the "Breakfast" category (Softia S).

Groups	Index	M ± S	M ± S (%)				p
		Day 1	Day 3	Day 5	Day 7	Day 14	
Thickener	Food consumption time, min	46.67 ± 3.96	44.27 ± 4.42 (−5.14)	41.40 ± 5.93 (−11.29)	41.73 ± 5.50 (−10.57)	39.73 ± 6.63 (−14.86)	<0.0001
Thickener	Number of chocks during fluid intake	13.47 ± 6.03	11.53 ± 5.69 (−14.36)	9.13 ± 5.74 (−32.18)	6.33 ± 5.33 (−52.97)	1.40 ± 1.80 (−89.60)	<0.0001
Thickener	Number of chocks after fluid intake	8.67 ± 4.50	7.73 ± 4.23 (−10.77)	6.20 ± 3.93 (−28.46)	4.67 ± 3.58 (−46.15)	0.53 ± 0.92 (−93.85)	<0.0001
Thickener	Calorie content	898.33 ± 123.12	847.17 ± 117.86 (−5.69)	778.87 ± 142.40 (−13.30)	782.87 ± 196.44 (−12.85)	784.67 ± 194.25 (−12.65)	0.1960
Thickener	P (proteins)	36.16 ± 11.57	38.56 ± 6.61 (6.65)	35.21 ± 8.94 (−2.61)	35.63 ± 12.40 (−1.46)	35.63 ± 12.40 (−1.46)	0.2171
Thickener	F (fats)	32.01 ± 7.27	30.29 ± 5.96 (−5.39)	26.69 ± 10.09 (−16.62)	27.37 ± 10.33 (−14.51)	27.37 ± 10.33 (−14.51)	0.3131
Thickener	C (carbohydrates)	103.19 ± 24.25	100.61 ± 24.16 (−2.50)	96.09 ± 16.59 (−6.88)	95.40 ± 22.82 (−7.56)	95.53 ± 22.58 (−7.43)	0.1363
Thickener	Amount of fluid intake	406.67 ± 25.26	404.00 ± 13.52 (−0.66)	414.67 ± 32.26 (1.97)	415.67 ± 28.59 (2.21)	417.33 ± 35.75 (2.62)	0.2708
Control	Food consumption time, min	44.27 ± 2.19	43.20 ± 2.08 (−2.41)	43.47 ± 2.56 (−1.81)	43.73 ± 2.91 (−1.20)	43.33 ± 3.62 (−2.11)	0.7084
Control	Number of chocks during fluid intake	14.80 ± 4.26	14.33 ± 4.37 (−3.15)	13.93 ± 4.25 (−5.86)	14.13 ± 4.60 (−4.50)	13.60 ± 5.07 (−8.11)	0.1298
Control	Number of chocks after fluid intake	11.13 ± 3.64	10.93 ± 3.99 (−1.80)	10.73 ± 3.77 (−3.59)	10.93 ± 4.15 (−1.80)	10.53 ± 4.41 (−5.39)	0.6015
Control	Calorie content	899.49 ± 176.08	834.33 ± 147.55 (−7.24)	804.50 ± 114.16 (−10.56)	890.00 ± 157.84 (−1.06)	890.00 ± 157.84 (−1.06)	0.5456
Control	P (proteins)	43.35 ± 11.33	39.44 ± 11.35 (−9.00)	38.05 ± 6.09 (−12.23)	41.84 ± 11.60 (−3.49)	41.37 ± 11.04 (−4.56)	0.0916
Control	F (fats)	34.75 ± 8.90	31.33 ± 6.98 (−9.84)	31.06 ± 7.60 (−10.63)	33.71 ± 7.64 (−3.00)	33.31 ± 7.55 (−4.15)	0.1444
Control	C (carbohydrates)	100.92 ± 21.81	94.93 ± 19.43 (−5.93)	90.07 ± 17.86 (−10.75)	102.55 ± 22.93 (1.61)	102.55 ± 22.93 (1.61)	0.7859
Control	Amount of fluid intake	417.33 ± 18.70	420.00 ± 20.70 (0.64)	421.33 ± 20.66 (0.96)	420.67 ± 19.44 (0.80)	402.67 ± 57.88 (−3.51)	0.4963

Statistically significant differences in indicators are highlighted in color, the p level is presented between the indicators "Day 1" and "Day 14."

Table 2.
Analysis of the dynamics of quantitative indicators for the "Lunch" category (Softia S).

Groups	Index	M ± S	M ± S (%)				p
		Day 1	Day 3	Day 5	Day 7	Day 14	
Thickener	Food consumption time, min	35.40 ± 5.04	35.47 ± 5.68 (0.19)	33.80 ± 6.57 (−4.52)	33.40 ± 6.09 (−5.65)	30.33 ± 6.18 (−14.31)	0.0098
Thickener	Number of chocks during fluid intake	9.40 ± 3.72	8.33 ± 3.89 (−11.35)	6.67 ± 3.96 (−29.08)	5.00 ± 3.53 (−46.81)	0.67 ± 0.90 (−92.91)	<0.0001
Thickener	Number of chocks after fluid intake	7.00 ± 3.05	5.87 ± 2.70 (−16.19)	4.73 ± 3.08 (−32.38)	3.80 ± 2.93 (−45.71)	0.21 ± 0.58 (−96.94)	<0.0001
Thickener	Calorie content	447.55 ± 54.75	496.98 ± 112.01 (11.05)	530.92 ± 79.63 (18.63)	448.04 ± 43.34 (0.11)	448.04 ± 43.34 (0.11)	0.0058
Thickener	P (proteins)	27.03 ± 4.83	30.49 ± 1.74 (12.78)	26.97 ± 3.31 (−0.25)	27.21 ± 3.36 (0.65)	27.21 ± 3.36 (0.65)	0.0186
Thickener	F (fats)	19.68 ± 4.44	21.82 ± 5.79 (10.87)	25.45 ± 3.11 (29.30)	22.74 ± 5.03 (15.52)	21.94 ± 5.38 (11.46)	0.1574
Thickener	C (carbohydrates)	38.26 ± 11.54	45.66 ± 13.33 (19.32)	44.67 ± 15.77 (16.75)	33.29 ± 11.11 (−13.01)	33.29 ± 11.11 (−13.00)	0.1551
Thickener	Amount of fluid intake	226.00 ± 22.30	226.00 ± 20.63 (0.00)	229.33 ± 17.10 (1.47)	219.33 ± 23.14 (−2.95)	213.33 ± 28.45 (−5.60)	0.1568
Control	Food consumption time, min	35.87 ± 3.46	33.67 ± 2.79 (−6.13)	34.47 ± 3.04 (−3.90)	34.33 ± 2.06 (−4.28)	32.87 ± 2.36 (−8.36)	0.0515
Control	Number of chocks during fluid intake	10.67 ± 2.55	9.87 ± 2.77 (−7.50)	10.47 ± 2.90 (−1.87)	10.27 ± 3.15 (−3.75)	10.47 ± 3.48 (−1.87)	0.0573
Control	Number of chocks after fluid intake	8.67 ± 2.79	8.20 ± 2.81 (−5.38)	8.60 ± 2.75 (−0.77)	8.47 ± 2.77 (−2.31)	8.67 ± 3.09 (0.00)	0.4334
Control	Calorie content	461.08 ± 66.18	536.11 ± 92.53 (16.27)	540.05 ± 86.38 (17.13)	438.73 ± 45.20 (−4.85)	438.78 ± 45.26 (−4.84)	0.0024
Control	P (proteins)	28.86 ± 3.03	29.58 ± 3.23 (2.50)	27.43 ± 3.82 (−4.95)	27.43 ± 3.31 (−4.93)	27.43 ± 3.31 (−4.93)	0.4098
Control	F (fats)	19.23 ± 3.56	23.18 ± 5.44 (20.50)	25.84 ± 4.12 (34.36)	20.73 ± 5.27 (7.78)	21.40 ± 4.25 (11.25)	0.0094
Control	C (carbohydrates)	40.77 ± 15.90	50.69 ± 16.18 (24.31)	46.89 ± 16.35 (15.00)	32.09 ± 9.64 (−21.29)	30.76 ± 10.63 (−24.56)	0.0015
Control	Amount of fluid intake	215.33 ± 15.06	214.67 ± 16.85 (−0.31)	213.33 ± 14.96 (−0.93)	213.33 ± 14.96 (−0.93)	218.00 ± 16.12 (1.24)	0.9375

Statistically significant differences in indicators are highlighted in color, the p level is presented between the indicators "Day 1" and "Day 14."

Table 3.
Analysis of the dynamics of quantitative indicators for the "Dinner" category (Softia S).

Groups	Numbers yes/no, Day 1	Increase/Decrease (%)				p
		Day 3–Day 1	Day 5–Day 1	Day 7–Day 1	Day 14–Day 1	
Thickener, breakfast	11/4	+2 (+50.0)/−1 (−9.1)	+2 (+50.0)/−2 (−18.2)	+2 (+50.0)/−4 (−36.4)	+0 (0.0)/−11 (−100.0)	0.0026
Control, breakfast	14/1	+0 (0.0)/−0 (0.0)	+0 (0.0)/−0 (0.0)	+0 (0.0)/−0 (0.0)	+0 (0.0)/−1 (−7.1)	10.000
Thickener, lunch	15/0	+0 (0.0)/−4 (−26.7)	+0 (0.0)/−4 (−26.7)	+0 (0.0)/−10 (−66.7)	+0 (0.0)/−14 (−93.3)	0.0005
Control, lunch	14/1	+0 (0.0)/−0 (0.0)	+0 (0.0)/−0 (0.0)	+0 (0.0)/−0 (0.0)	+0 (0.0)/−1 (−7.1)	10.000
Thickener, dinner	12/3	+0 (0.0)/−3 (−25.0)	+1 (+33.3)/−7 (−58.3)	+2 (+66.7)/−9 (−75.0)	+0 (0.0)/−12 (−100.0)	0.0015
Control, dinner	14/1	+0 (0.0)/−0 (0.0)	+0 (0.0)/−0 (0.0)	+0 (0.0)/−0 (0.0)	+0 (0.0)/−1 (−7.1)	10.000

Statistically significant differences in indicators are highlighted in color, the p level is presented between the indicators "Day 1" and "Day 14."

Table 4.
Analysis of the dynamics of quality indicators (Softia S).

G. On the 1st, 14th, and 28th days of the study, the patients underwent a blood test, determining the level of prealbumin and urea in the blood serum. Furthermore, the patients were examined daily by a speech therapist and a nutritionist. During the daily assessment, the amount of food consumed orally (kcal), the amount of oral nutritional support performed (kcal), the content of proteins, fats, and carbohydrates of the food consumed, the amount of choking during or after drinking, body temperature (number of cases of pyrexia), the presence of dysphonia with phlegm (hoarse/hoarse voice if phlegm is present) are assessed. In addition, we assessed body weight every 2 weeks. The study of the product Softia G included 15 patients, including 8 men and 7 women, with the following distribution:

- By age: four patients—from 73 to 79 years old, five patients—from 63 to 69 years old, four patients—from 45 to 47 years old, two patients—from 22 to 39 years old;
- By pathology: traumatic brain injury (TBI)—2, cerebrovascular accident (CVA)—13.

According to the initial speech therapy evaluation, all patients had a mild degree of dysphagia, making it unnecessary to place a tracheostomy and insert a nasogastric tube for feeding. Moreover, the selected patients, according to the Rosenbek scale (PAS), had an aspiration rating of 2 (food enters the airways, remains above the vocal cords, and clears his throat from the airway), according to the Fiberoptic Endoscopic Dysphagia Severity Scale (FEDSS) scale, all—a penetration rating of 3 (fluid penetration with good protective reflex).

According to the speech therapy examination data, by the end of the study, nine patients showed a complete recovery of the swallowing function, six patients retained residual effects in mild choking (no significant changes were noted outside the use of the product).

During the first 14 days of observation (without *Softia G*), there was no significant increase in food intake. After introducing Softia G into the diet of patients, there was

Groups	Index	M ± S	M ± S (%)				p
		Day 1	Day 3	Day 5	Day 7	Day 14	
Thickener	The amount of food consumed, kcal	320.13 ± 62.22	354.27 ± 109.48 (10.66)	388.47 ± 89.01 (21.35)	463.27 ± 94.30 (44.71)	532.60 ± 111.39 (66.37)	0.0010
Thickener	Number of chocks during fluid intake	9.87 ± 3.48	8.20 ± 3.00 (−16.89%)	6.20 ± 2.78 (−37.16%)	4.40 ± 2.20 (−55.41%)	1.20 ± 1.70 (−87.84%)	<0.0001
Thickener	Number of chocks after fluid intake	8.33 ± 3.27	6.87 ± 3.02 (−17.60%)	5.13 ± 2.42 (−38.40%)	3.53 ± 1.81 (−57.60%)	0.73 ± 1.03 (−91.20%)	<0.0001
Thickener	P (proteins)	11.93 ± 4.22	14.27 ± 5.62 (19.55)	14.13 ± 5.22 (18.44)	15.80 ± 3.93 (32.40)	18.20 ± 4.31 (52.51)	0.0276
Thickener	F (fats)	11.87 ± 3.31	15.13 ± 4.07 (27.53)	14.07 ± 4.03 (18.54)	18.40 ± 4.73 (55.06)	21.13 ± 5.79 (78.09)	0.0021
Thickener	C (carbohydrates)	41.93 ± 8.62	41.20 ± 17.72 (−1.75)	51.00 ± 11.05 (21.62)	59.00 ± 12.36 (40.70)	67.67 ± 13.67 (61.37)	<0.0001
Control	The amount of food consumed, kcal	309.00 ± 75.28	336.87 ± 63.51 (9.02)	292.73 ± 58.80 (−5.26)	324.73 ± 75.18 (5.09)	356.60 ± 72.81 (15.40)	0.1135
Control	Number of chocks during fluid intake	9.47 ± 3.81	9.53 ± 3.07 (0.70)	10.07 ± 3.26 (6.34)	9.67 ± 3.22 (2.11)	9.80 ± 3.30 (3.52)	0.4692
Control	Number of chocks after fluid intake	8.33 ± 3.52	8.00 ± 3.02 (−4.00)	9.00 ± 3.02 (8.00)	8.40 ± 3.29 (0.80)	8.67 ± 2.82 (4.00)	0.3376
Control	P (proteins)	12.73 ± 4.13	13.93 ± 3.24 (9.42)	11.33 ± 2.77 (−10.99)	12.33 ± 3.09 (−3.14)	12.80 ± 2.81 (−0.52)	0.1389
Control	F (fats)	11.13 ± 4.21	13.93 ± 3.28 (25.15)	10.27 ± 2.94 (−7.78)	12.67 ± 4.06 (13.77)	13.93 ± 4.27 (25.15)	0.1355
Control	C (carbohydrates)	39.20 ± 9.35	38.27 ± 11.29 (−2.38)	38.93 ± 8.84 (−0.68)	40.40 ± 9.43 (3.06)	44.07 ± 8.60 (12.41)	0.3772

Statistically significant differences in indicators are highlighted in color, the p level is presented between the indicators "Day 1" and "Day 14."

Table 5.
Analysis of the dynamics of quantitative indicators for the "Breakfast" category (Softia G).

Groups	Index	M ± S	M ± S (%)				P
		Day 1	Day 3	Day 5	Day 7	Day 14	
Thickener	The amount of food consumed, kcal	463.80 ± 143.57	499.33 ± 135.98 (7.66)	473.93 ± 109.50 (2.18)	555.80 ± 103.80 (19.84)	643.40 ± 83.55 (38.72)	0.0024
Thickener	Number of chocks during fluid intake	15.73 ± 5.56	13.93 ± 6.11 (−11.44)	11.13 ± 5.66 (−29.24)	8.40 ± 5.21 (−46.61)	2.33 ± 3.52 (−85.17)	<0.0001
Thickener	Number of chocks after fluid intake	12.60 ± 5.79	10.80 ± 6.55 (−14.29)	8.67 ± 5.50 (−31.22)	6.93 ± 4.45 (−44.97)	1.60 ± 2.75 (−87.30)	<0.0001
Thickener	P (proteins)	17.13 ± 5.22	18.80 ± 4.97 (9.73)	19.13 ± 3.31 (11.67)	21.33 ± 2.41 (24.51)	25.40 ± 2.35 (48.25)	<0.0001
Thickener	F (fats)	18.20 ± 6.14	21.53 ± 9.31 (18.32)	17.27 ± 5.66 (−5.13)	17.60 ± 5.77 (−3.30)	21.13 ± 6.63 (16.12)	0.0768
Thickener	C (carbohydrates)	53.33 ± 24.42	62.20 ± 20.71 (16.63)	61.27 ± 15.41 (14.88)	73.93 ± 9.87 (38.63)	88.20 ± 8.23 (65.38)	<0.0001
Control	The amount of food consumed, kcal	357.53 ± 105.37	358.93 ± 94.52 (0.39)	269.40 ± 90.68 (−24.65)	298.33 ± 92.58 (−16.56)	301.87 ± 89.63 (−15.57)	0.0983
Control	Number of chocks during fluid intake	16.33 ± 6.66	15.60 ± 5.88 (−4.49)	16.20 ± 5.68 (−0.82)	15.67 ± 5.22 (−4.08)	15.80 ± 5.95 (−3.27)	0.5060
Control	Number of chocks after fluid intake	13.80 ± 7.01	13.33 ± 6.16 (−3.38)	13.80 ± 5.95 (0.00)	13.47 ± 5.44 (−2.42)	13.13 ± 5.96 (−4.83)	0.4799
Control	P (proteins)	13.40 ± 3.68	13.93 ± 3.58 (3.98)	11.13 ± 3.52 (−16.92)	11.47 ± 3.48 (−14.43)	11.80 ± 3.10 (−11.94)	0.1165
Control	F (fats)	14.53 ± 4.44	14.20 ± 4.35 (−2.29)	9.93 ± 4.42 (−31.65)	10.33 ± 4.39 (−28.90)	10.73 ± 4.57 (−26.15)	0.0468
Control	C (carbohydrates)	43.40 ± 13.39	43.60 ± 11.26 (0.46)	33.60 ± 11.24 (−22.58)	36.80 ± 11.51 (−15.21)	37.93 ± 10.46 (−12.60)	0.0816

Statistically significant differences in indicators are highlighted in color, the p level is presented between the indicators "Day 1" and "Day 14."

Table 6.
Analysis of the dynamics of quantitative indicators for the "Lunch" category (Softia G).

Groups	Index	M ± S	M ± S (%)				p
		Day 1	Day 3	Day 5	Day 7	Day 14	
Thickener	The amount of food consumed, kcal	356.00 ± 82.37	426.80 ± 133.60 (19.89)	499.13 ± 107.84 (40.21)	504.20 ± 85.97 (41.63)	530.53 ± 69.18 (49.03)	0.0056
Thickener	Number of chocks during fluid intake	10.00 ± 3.16	7.80 ± 3.45 (−22.00)	6.47 ± 2.75 (−35.33)	5.07 ± 3.97 (−49.33)	1.13 ± 1.64 (−88.67)	<0.0001
Thickener	Number of chocks after fluid intake	8.60 ± 2.92	6.40 ± 2.90 (−25.58)	5.20 ± 2.37 (−39.53)	3.53 ± 2.26 (−58.91)	0.73 ± 1.16 (−91.47)	<0.0001
Thickener	P (proteins)	17.20 ± 5.28	21.93 ± 4.99 (27.52)	24.00 ± 4.71 (39.53)	27.20 ± 4.21 (58.14)	28.93 ± 4.43 (68.22)	<0.0001
Thickener	F (fats)	16.00 ± 4.87	19.07 ± 6.95 (19.17)	21.20 ± 4.09 (32.50)	20.47 ± 5.71 (27.92)	21.40 ± 4.97 (33.75)	0.0942
Thickener	C (carbohydrates)	35.33 ± 8.54	41.07 ± 14.99 (16.23)	51.27 ± 18.85 (45.09)	52.33 ± 9.86 (48.11)	55.13 ± 8.80 (56.04)	0.0006
Control	The amount of food consumed, kcal	278.07 ± 79.93	292.67 ± 74.94 (5.25)	317.33 ± 77.43 (14.12)	305.47 ± 79.86 (9.85)	251.67 ± 68.26 (−9.49)	0.2569
Control	Number of chocks during fluid intake	9.80 ± 3.21	9.47 ± 3.25 (−3.40)	9.87 ± 3.29 (0.68)	9.47 ± 3.04 (−3.40)	9.80 ± 3.34 (0.00)	0.4647
Control	Number of chocks after fluid intake	8.47 ± 3.25	8.33 ± 2.94 (−1.57)	8.27 ± 3.13 (−2.36)	8.13 ± 3.11 (−3.94)	9.13 ± 3.25 (7.87)	0.2949
Control	P (proteins)	13.73 ± 4.61	14.07 ± 3.01 (2.43)	16.80 ± 5.25 (22.33)	16.73 ± 5.64 (21.84)	13.53 ± 3.94 (−1.46)	0.2139
Control	F (fats)	12.33 ± 5.08	12.00 ± 4.86 (−2.70)	14.07 ± 3.99 (14.05)	12.53 ± 3.80 (1.62)	10.73 ± 4.33 (−12.97)	0.3589
Control	C (carbohydrates)	29.73 ± 9.58	33.47 ± 10.90 (12.56)	31.13 ± 9.46 (4.71)	32.13 ± 9.45 (8.07)	26.73 ± 8.10 (−10.09)	0.4474

Statistically significant differences in indicators are highlighted in color, the p level is presented between the indicators "Day 1" and "Day 14."

Table 7.
Analysis of the dynamics of quantitative indicators for the "Dinner" category (Softia G).

Groups	Numbers yes/no, Day 1	Increase/decrease (%)				p
		Day 3–Day 1	Day 5–Day 1	Day 7–Day 1	Day 14–Day 1	
Thickener, breakfast	8/7	0 (0.0)/−3 (−37.5)	0 (0.0)/−6 (−75.0)	0 (0.0)/−8 (−100.0)	0 (0.0)/−8 (−100.0)	0.0133
Control, breakfast	8/7	0 (0.0)/0 (0.0)	0 (0.0)/0 (0.0)	0 (0.0)/0 (0.0)	0 (0.0)/0 (0.0)	10.000
Thickener, lunch	8/7	0 (0.0)/−3 (−37.5)	0 (0.0)/−6 (−75.0)	0 (0.0)/−6 (−75.0)	0 (0.0)/−8 (−100.0)	0.0133
Control, lunch	8/7	0 (0.0)/0 (0.0)	0 (0.0)/0 (0.0)	0 (0.0)/0 (0.0)	0 (0.0)/0 (0.0)	10.000
Thickener, dinner	8/7	0 (0.0)/−2 (−25.0)	0 (0.0)/−7 (−87.5)	0 (0.0)/−8 (−100.0)	0 (0.0)/−8 (−100.0)	0.0133
Control, dinner	8/7	0 (0.0)/0 (0.0)	0 (0.0)/0 (0.0)	0 (0.0)/0 (0.0)	0 (0.0)/0 (0.0)	10.000

Statistically significant differences in indicators are highlighted in color, the p level is presented between the indicators "Day 1" and "Day 14."

Table 8.
Analysis of the dynamics of quality indicators (Softia G).

a consumption increment in the amount of food both once (during one meal) and daily. Laboratory values during the observation period were relatively stable.

For statistical analysis, the stage without using a thickener was designated as "Control group," the stage with the use of this product as "Thickener Group." To test the hypothesis about significant changes—the periods of "Day 1," "Day 3," "Day 5," "Day 7," and "Day 14" were statistically analyzed. Six out of 12 indicators in the "Breakfast" category during the period under review had statistically significant changes. The most significant changes are found for the indicators in the thickener group: "Number of chocks after fluid intake" (an average of 7.6 min; $p < 0.0001$); "the Number of chocks during fluid intake" (average of 8.7 min; $p < 0.0001$); "the food consumption time" (an average of 26.5 min; $p < 0.0001$). Whereas, the tiniest changes between periods are observed in the following indicators in the control group: "The number of gasps after hydration", "C (fats)" and "The number of chocks during fluid intake" ($p > 0.0001$). (see **Table 5**).

Six out of 12 indicators in the "Lunch" category had statistically significant changes during the time under review. The most significant changes are found for the indicator in the thickener group: "Number of chocks during fluid intake" (average 13.4; $p < 0.0001$); indicator "C (fats)" (average of 34.9; $p < 0.0001$); indicator "P (proteins)," (average 8.3; $p < 0.0001$). The few changes between periods are observed in the following indicators: "P (proteins), in the control group," "The number of chocks after fluid intake, control," and "The number of chocks during fluid intake, control" ($p > 0.0001$) (**Table 6**).

During the time under review, five out of 12 indicators in the "Dinner" category had statistically significant changes. The most significant changes are found for the indicator: "Number of chocks after fluid intake, the thickener" (average of 7.9; $p < 0.0001$); indicator "Number of chocks during fluid intake, the thickener" (an average of 8.9; $p < 0.0001$); indicator "P (proteins), the thickener" (average 11.7; $p < 0.0001$). The few changes between periods are observed in the following indicators: "F (fats), in control," "C (carbohydrates), in control," and "The number of chocks during fluid intake, in control" ($p > 0.0001$) (**Table 7**).

DOI: http://dx.doi.org/10.5772/intechopen.101798

When we assessed the changes in the qualitative indicator (the presence or absence of dysphonia with sputum), we found out that there were statistically significant differences in the dynamics of dysphonia from the 1st to the 14th day of the study in the primary group during all meals. In contrast, no significant differences were present in the control group (**Table 8**).

5. Discussion

The thickening products have found wide applications in our practice. An option for a household-friendly thickener expands the possibilities for adequate oral fluid intake. Earlier, in treating and preventing dysphagia, starch was used to thicken liquids (fruit jelly, milk jelly), which had several disadvantages: the need for thermal processing and the difficulty of dosing the degree of thickening. Currently, many specialized thickeners are easy to use and adjust the required degree of thickening. One of them is the reviewed product *Softia S* of NUTRI company, which allows thickening of any liquid, including drinking water, without changing the organoleptic properties of the drink.

The use of this product facilitated the fluid intake by patients after stroke and TBI with mild dysphagia when swallowing is complicated. Therefore, the use of the product has led to significant facilitation of patient care by medical staff and optimization of their working hours. Furthermore, the regular use of the product decreased the degree of dysphagia resulting from the normalizing act of swallowing due to the training of the oropharyngeal phase in conditions of collective work of the oral-articulatory apparatus, the muscles of the larynx; also, reducing the time of eating, reducing the frequency of choking and manifestations of dysphonia with sputum contributed to an improvement in the quality of life of patients and the effectiveness of rehabilitation measures.

It is difficult to achieve a uniform consistency of mashed products at home. Often, patients take factory-made and ready-made baby purees. Although, on the one hand, this somewhat limits the choice of flavor combinations, on the other, it significantly increases the financial burden on the patient's family. Therefore, we considered the possibility of using the product *Softia G* from NUTRI.

This product made it easier for patients to take food after stroke and TBI with mild dysphagia and difficulty swallowing food, which has led to significant ease of patient care by medical personnel and, most importantly, increased the amount of food consumed.

The degree of dysphagia decreased with regular use of the product, as in the above-considered option for thickening drinks, due to the oropharyngeal phase training in conditions of the oral-articulatory collective work apparatus and the muscles of the larynx.

The frequency of choking and manifestations of dysphonia with sputum decreased significantly, contributing to an improvement in the quality of life of patients and the effectiveness of rehabilitation measures. In addition, an increase in the consumption of macronutrients and the total amount of food received helps prevent the development of protein-energy malnutrition due to underfeeding and improve the nutritional status of patients.

Providing oral food and drink intake in patients with mild dysphagia of various origins is of great importance both in the process of rehabilitation and in subsequent care. It is necessary, if possible, to strive to obtain the total amount of nutrition through natural routes in this category of patients. For these purposes, the use of thickeners *Softia S* and *Softia G* is suitable. The inclusion of these products in the diet increases the safety of oral intake of food and liquids for patients, increases the amount of food eaten, and can also help to eliminate the phenomena of mild dysphagia during rehabilitation.

6. Ready-made dense enteral feeding mixtures

Along with the use of thickeners in the clinical practice of nutritional support in dysphagia, ready-made dense enteral nutrition mixtures are now widely used:

- grade 1: syrup consistency; it can be drunk through a straw or from a cup, a thin layer remains on the walls
- grade 2: honey consistency; it can be drunk from a cup, a thick layer remains on the walls.
- grade 3: yogurt consistency; cannot be drunk, but we can eat with a spoon
- grade 4: consistency of thick sour cream, in which the spoon can stand on the mixture.

The positive aspect of these mixtures is, first of all, the fact that they are completely ready for use and do not require additional costs. In addition, they have good palatability based on patient preferences, are easy to use by patients, meet the needs with a minimum amount of nutrition, and maintain compliance with therapy. They are mainly high in calories (over 1.2 kcal/ml) and protein. The stable consistency of the mixtures corresponds to the adaptation of food and liquid by the type and degree of swallowing disorders. The use of ready-made mixtures is currently one of the most common medical recommendations. According to the literature, over 80% of physicians consider the intake of thickened liquids to be the most effective therapeutic strategy. One of the reasons for the widespread use of ready-made mixtures is that thickened mixtures do not require adequate cognitive and linguistic abilities. Therefore, the use of such mixtures increases the effectiveness of nutritional support [15, 32–34].

7. Conclusion

Neurogenic dysphagia is a multidimensional and multifactorial problem. This syndrome is typical for many conditions with different etiology, pathogenic mechanisms, and predictable outcomes. Therefore, it is essential to select an adequate nutritional therapy, considering all the patient's characteristics. Each of the described approaches has advantages and limitations. The choice of nutritional support method depends on the degree of dysphagia, the structure of the neurological disease, and short- and long-term prognosis. Patients with mild dysphagia, especially with progressive neurological diseases, should initially be offered ready-made dense enteral feeding mixtures or specialized thickeners, according to the recommendations of a speech therapist. Acute patients with severe-to-moderate dysphagia should be fed with a nasogastric tube. If, in the next 4 weeks, a transition to *per os* feeding is not expected, a gastrostomy is required. However, we recommend that you do not overstretch with the PEG. In the process of rehabilitation, it is effective to combine nutrition through a gastrostomy tube and training of feeding through the mouth with the use of thickeners or ready-made nutritional mixtures.

Funding source

The studies *Softia S* and *Softia G* were carried out with the financial support of the Ministry of Agriculture, Forestry and Fisheries of Japan.

Conflict of interest

Financial support of the studies *Softia S* and *Softia G* was provided by the Ministry of Agriculture, Forestry and Fisheries of Japan; NUTRI participated in the design of the studies *Softia S* and *Softia G* and discussion of the results.

Author details

Marina V. Petrova[1,2], Alexandr E. Shestopalov[1,3], Alexandra V. Yakovleva[1], Pranil Pradhan[1] and Alexey A. Yakovlev[1]*

1 Federal Research and Clinical Center of Intensive Care Medicine and Rehabilitology, Moscow, Russia

2 Peoples' Friendship University of Russia (RUDN University), Moscow, Russia

3 Federal State Budgetary Educational Institution of Further Professional Education "Russian Medical Academy of Continuous Professional Education" of the Ministry of Healthcare of the Russian Federation, Moscow, Russia

*Address all correspondence to: avyakovleva@fnkcrr.ru

References

[1] Sabbouh T, Torbey MT. Malnutrition in Stroke Patients: Risk Factors, Assessment, and Management. Neurocritical Care. 2018;**29**(3):374-384. DOI: 10.1007/s12028-017-0436-1

[2] Turley R, Cohen S. Impact of voice and swallowing problems in the elderly. Otolaryngology and Head and Neck Surgery. 2009;**140**(1):33-36. DOI: 10.1016/j.otohns.2008.10.010

[3] Holland G, Jayasekeran V, Pendleton N, et al. Prevalence and symptom profiling of oropharyngeal dysphagia in a community dwelling of an elderly population: A self-reporting questionnaire survey. Diseases of the Esophagus. 2011;**24**(7):476-480. DOI: 10.1111/j.1442-2050.2011.01182.x

[4] Lin LC, Wu SC, Chen HS, et al. Prevalence of impaired swallowing in institutionalized older people in Taiwan. Journal of the American Geriatrics Society. 2002;**50**(6):1118-1123. DOI: 10.1046/j.1532-5415.2002.50270.x

[5] Stakhovskaya LV, Melnikova EV, editors. Diagnosis and treatment of dysphagia in diseases of the central nervous system: Clinical recommendations. Moscow; 2013. Available from: https://rehabrus.ru/Docs/2020/Disfagia_last.pdf

[6] Vidal Casariego A, Suárez Silva C, Lugo Rodríguez G, Pita Gutiérrez F, Almeida Seoane MC, Rodríguez Ramos MJ, et al. Utility of the EAT-10 in the detection of dysphagia in high-risk hospitalisation units at a university hospital: A cross-sectional study. Nutrición Hospitalaria. 2020;**37**(6):1197-1200. DOI: 10.20960/nh.03233

[7] Ivashkin VT, Mayev IV, Trukhmanov AS, et al. Diagnostics and treatment of dysphagia: Clinical guidelines of the Russian gastroenterological association. Russian Journal of Gastroenterology, Hepatology, and Coloproctology. 2015;**25**(5):84-93

[8] Mansare ML, Kouda DA, Diallo IM, Bakhoum M, Mourabit S, Toure K, et al. What is the nutritional status of your patients suffering from strokes. Revue Neurologique (Paris). 2020;**176**(5):366-369. DOI: 10.1016/j.neurol.2019.09.009

[9] Özpak Akkuş Ö, Mermer M, Hamdanoğullari D, Erden B. Does nutritional treatment in patients with dysphagia affect malnutrition and anxiety? Nutrición Hospitalaria. 2021;**38**(3):533-539. DOI: 10.20960/nh.03430

[10] Reverberi C, Lombardi F, Lusuardi M, Pratesi A, Di Bari M. Development of the decannulation prediction tool in patients with dysphagia after acquired brain injury. Journal of the American Medical Directors Association. 2019;**20**(4):470-475.e1. DOI: 10.1016/j.jamda.2018.09.022

[11] Schwarz M, Coccetti A, Murdoch A, Cardell E. The impact of aspiration pneumonia and nasogastric feeding on clinical outcomes in stroke patients: A retrospective cohort study. Journal of Clinical Nursing. 2018;**27**(1-2):e235-e241. DOI: 10.1111/jocn.13922

[12] Warnecke T, Im S, Kaiser C, Hamacher C, Oelenberg S, Dziewas R. Aspiration and dysphagia screening in acute stroke—The Gugging Swallowing Screen revisited. European Journal of Neurology. 2017;**24**(4):594-601. DOI: 10.1111/ene.13251

[13] Ho CH, Lin WC, Hsu YF, Lee IH, Hung YC. One-year risk of pneumonia and mortality in patients with poststroke dysphagia: A nationwide population-based study. Journal of Stroke and Cerebrovascular Diseases. 2018;**27**(5):1311-1317. DOI: 10.1016/j.jstrokecerebrovasdis.2017.12.017

[14] Kim H, Suh Y. Changes in the dysphagia and nutritional status of patients with brain injury. Journal of Clinical Nursing. 2018;**27**(7-8):1581-1588. DOI: 10.1111/jocn.14226

[15] Ballesteros Pomar MD, Palazuelo AL. How is the patient's nutrition after a stroke? Nutrición Hospitalaria. 2017;**34**(Suppl. 1):46-56. DOI: 10.20960/nh.1239

[16] Burgos R, Bretón I, Cereda E, Desport JC, Dziewas R, Genton L, et al. ESPEN guideline clinical nutrition in neurology. Clinical Nutrition. 2018;**37**(1):354-396. DOI: 10.1016/j.clnu.2017.09.003

[17] Diendéré J, Millogo A, Preux PM, Jésus P, Desport JC. Changes in nutritional state and dysphagia in stroke patients monitored during a 14-d period in a Burkina Faso hospital setting. Nutrition. 2018;**48**:55-60. DOI: 10.1016/j.nut.2017.10.022

[18] Fernández Martínez P, Barajas Galindo DE, Arés Luque A, Rodríguez Sánchez E, Ballesteros-Pomar MD. Clinical repercussions of dysphagia and malnutrition in the stroke patient. Endocrinology, Diabetes and Nutrition. 2018;**65**(10):625-626. DOI: 10.1016/j.endinu.2018.05.013

[19] Ramos-Vázquez AG, Reyes-Torres CA, Castillo-Martínez L, Serralde Zúñiga AE. Body composition by bioelectrical impedance, muscle strength, and nutritional risk in oropharyngeal dysphagia patients. Nutrición Hospitalaria. 2021;**38**(2):315-320. DOI: 10.20960/nh.03374

[20] Jaul E, Factor H, Karni S, Schiffmiller T, Meiron O. Spasticity and dementia increase the risk of pressure ulcers. International Wound Journal. 2019;**16**(3):847-851

[21] Magny E, Vallet H, Cohen-Bittan J, Raux M, Meziere A, Verny M, et al. Pressure ulcers are associated with 6-month mortality in elderly patients with hip fracture managed in orthogeriatric care pathway. Archives of Osteoporosis. 29 Aug 2017;**12**(1):77

[22] Schott M, Golin A, de Jesus SR, Alves BP, Dachi L, Cassol MC, et al. Dysphagia, immobility, and diet acceptance: Main factors associated with increased risk of pressure injury in patients hospitalized after stroke. Advances in Skin & Wound Care. 2020;**33**(10):527-532. DOI: 10.1097/01.ASW.0000694140.54146.75

[23] Yakovlev AA, Shulutko AM, Osmanov JG, Yakovleva AV, Natroshvili AG, Nasirov FN, et al. Objectification of the choice of treatment tactics for decubital ulcers in patients in chronic critical illness due to brain damage. Moscow Surgical Journal. 2020;**2**(72):90-96. DOI: 10.17238/issn2072-3180.2020.2.90-96

[24] Mañas-Martínez AB, Bucar-Barjud M, Campos-Fernández J, Gimeno-Orna JA, Pérez-Calvo J, Ocón-Bretón J. Association of positive screening for dysphagia with nutritional status and long-term mortality in hospitalized elderly patients. Endocrinology, Diabetes and Nutrition. 2018;**65**(7):402-408. DOI: 10.1016/j.endinu.2018.02.004

[25] Juan W, Zhen H, Yan-Ying F, Hui-Xian Y, Tao Z, Pei-Fen G, et al. A comparative study of two tube feeding methods in patients with dysphagia after stroke: A randomized controlled trial. Journal of Stroke and Cerebrovascular Diseases. 2020;**29**(3):104602. DOI: 10.1016/j.jstrokecerebrovasdis.2019.104602

[26] Kim G, Baek S, Park HW, Kang EK, Lee G. Effect of nasogastric tube on aspiration risk: Results from 147 patients with dysphagia and literature review. Dysphagia. 2018;**33**(6):731-738. DOI: 10.1007/s00455-018-9894-7

[27] Wang ZY, Chen JM, Ni GX. Effect of an indwelling nasogastric tube on swallowing function in elderly post-stroke dysphagia patients with long-term nasal feeding. BMC Neurology. 2019;**19**(1):83. DOI: 10.1186/s12883-019-1314-6

[28] Wu CC, Huang HH, Lin HH, Chang WK. Oropharyngeal dysphagia increased the risk of pneumonia in patients undergoing nasogastric tube feeding. Asia Pacific Journal of Clinical Nutrition. 2020;**29**(2):266-273. DOI: 10.6133/apjcn.202007_29(2).0009

[29] Patita M, Nunes G, Grunho M, Santos CA, Fonseca J. Endoscopic gastrostomy for nutritional support in post-stroke dysphagia. Nutrición Hospitalaria . 9 Dec 2021;**38**(6):1126-1131

[30] WGO Global Guidelines. Practical recommendations of the World Gastroenterological Organization "Dysphagia". World Gastroenterology Organisation; 2014. Available from: http://www.worldgastroenterology.org/UserFiles/file/guidelines/dysphagia-russian-2014.pdf

[31] Ojo O, Brooke J. The use of enteral nutrition in the management of stroke. Nutrients. 2016;**8**(12):827. DOI: 10.3390/nu8120827

[32] Śledzik A, Szlendak P. Dysphagia in neurological disorders. Wiadomości Lekarskie. 2020;**73**(9 cz. 1):1848-1852

[33] Gong L, Wang Y, Shi J. Enteral nutrition management in stroke patients: A narrative review. Annals of Palliative Medicine. 2021;**10**(10):11191-11202. DOI: 10.21037/apm-21-2922

[34] Shimazu S, Yoshimura Y, Kudo M, Nagano F, Bise T, Shiraishi A, et al. Frequent and personalized nutritional support leads to improved nutritional status, activities of daily living, and dysphagia after stroke. Nutrition. 2021;**83**:111091. DOI: 10.1016/j.nut.2020.111091

Chapter 6

Surgical Treatment of Esophageal Advanced Achalasia

José Luis Braga de Aquino
and Vânia Aparecida Leandro-Merhi

Abstract

Of the several procedures that has to treat esophageal achalasia, the esophagectomy is to be the most indicated in advanced disease, which prompted Pinotti the disseminate the transmediastinal esophagectomy technique in the 1970s, with the advantage of avoiding thoracotomy. Nevertheless, several series demonstrated that this technique was not exempt from complications one of which could lead to massive hemopneumothorax due to injury to the trachea- bronchial tree and vessels due the periesophagitis that may be present with consequent adherence of the esophagus to these noble organs. Thus, Aquino in 1996 introduced the esophageal mucosectomy technique with preservation of the esophageal muscle tunic at the level of mediastinum as well as the transposition of the stomach to the cervical region inside in this tunic for the reconstruction of digestive tract. The advantage of this procedure is to avoid transgression of the mediastinum. This author describes in details this procedure, and shows early results and late evaluation using the ECKARDT score in a series of patients showing the advantages of the esophageal mucosectomy due the low incidence of immediate postoperative complications and good resolution in long term due the absence of symptoms in most patients.

Keywords: Advanced achalasia, Chagasic megaesophagus, Esophageal achalasia, Esophageal mucosectomy, Esophagectomy

1. Introduction

Achalasia is one of the most studied affections associated with esophageal motility and is characterized by incomplete relaxation of the lower esophageal sphincter and absence of peristalsis along the esophageal body. Consequently, the food transit towards the stomach becomes hampered, which makes the patient present dysphagia as the main symptom. Other symptoms such as regurgitation of saliva and undigested food, heartburn, chest pain and respiratory symptoms such as nocturnal cough, recurrent aspiration and pneumonia have also been reported [1, 2].

The incidence of achalasia is similar in most countries, ranging from 0.7 to 1.6 per 100,000 inhabitants/year and with a prevalence of 1.8 to 12.6 per 100,000 inhabitants [2, 3].

Although idiopathic achalasia and Chagas disease have different etiologies, both conditions have, in fact, the same clinical, radiological, endoscopic and manometric presentation [1–3].

2. Achalasia therapeutics

Different methods have been proposed for the treatment of this condition, none of which seems to be optimal, as they do not act directly on the pathophysiology of the disease [1, 4, 5]. Thus, the main objective this disease treatment is to rescue swallowing and diagnose potential diseases that may occur in the dilated esophagus, consequent to long lasting food stasis.

Extramucosal cardiomyotomy, with its different technical variants, remains the most widely used surgical procedure, and with the advent of minimally invasive surgery today, the endoscopic (POEM) or laparoscopic approach has been widely accepted [2–7].

The good results obtained in myotomy using the minimally invasive technique are for cases of non-advanced achalasia, corresponding to an esophageal diameter that does not exceed 6 cm and that in high-resolution manometry reveals type II Chicago classification [2–4]. This has recently been well demonstrated in a meta-analysis involving 1575 patients with achalasia type II, submitted to laparoscopic myotomy with fundoplication with medium and long-term follow-up, that demonstrated a success rate with adequate rescue of swallowing in 92% of patients [8]. These results confirm what has been previously demonstrated by other authors who made assessments 1 to 18 years after surgery, in a compilation of 39 series with 3,086 patients with non-advanced achalasia undergoing this surgical procedure, who presented an average of 89% of excellent results [9].

Although laparoscopic myotomy is considered the first-line treatment for non-advanced achalasia, it is an invasive procedure though, that requires general anesthesia, which can lead to greater morbidity in the immediate postoperative period, especially in patients with unsatisfactory cardiopulmonary clinical conditions [2, 4, 10].

This is the reason for the advent of endoscopic myotomy, a procedure described by the Japanese school, and which consists, in the realization, under endoscopic vision, of a long extension submucosal tunnel from the end of the middle esophagus to 2 cm below the columnar squamous junction, in order to expose and section more adequately the esophagus circular muscle fibers [11]. The great advantage of this procedure is to minimize the surgical trauma that can potentially occur with more intensity through the laparoscopic approach [2–4, 12].

Some series have shown in a mean 3-year follow-up after surgery that endoscopic myotomy is comparable in terms of good results to 87 to 93% with the laparoscopic route results when evaluated by the ECKARDT score, thus providing good quality of life in patients with non-advanced achalasia [4, 13–16].

Although endoscopic myotomy has the advantage of avoiding further surgical trauma, in an evaluation carried out in the medium and long term, it has been shown, however, that endoscopic myotomy predisposes to greater gastroesophageal reflux when compared to laparoscopic myotomy, since in the latter a partial fundoplication surgery is performed. This has recently been shown in meta-analysis studies with pH monitoring. It was found that the rate of acid exposure can range from 39 to 58% after endoscopic myotomy decreasing to only 7.6% to 16.8% when compared to surgical myotomy [17, 18].

Although surgical/endoscopic myotomy demonstrates good results in the adequate rescue of swallowing in patients with non-advanced achalasia, this is not evidenced though in patients who have this condition with an esophagus diameter greater than 6 cm and in high-resolution manometry having a type I Chicago classification, due to the lack of adequate contractility of the entire esophagus, as has been shown recently [2–4].

Thus, other authors began to standardize cardioplasty procedures for patients with advanced achalasia, in order to promote a more adequate esophageal emptying, mainly by the techniques described by Thal et al., 1965, Hatafuku et al. in 1972, and Serra Doria et al. in 1968, with the experience of the Brazilian surgical school being outstanding, since in this country, advanced achalasia is quite frequent, due to the predominance of the Chagas etiology [19–22].

However, mid-term studies have shown that cardioplasties have not always yielded satisfactory results, mainly due to the difficulty in emptying the esophagus, and due to the gastroesophageal reflux that such procedure can trigger [20, 22–24]. This fact has been well demonstrated more recently by Aquino et al. [25], who evaluated the 5 years late postoperative period in 19 patients with recurrent advanced achalasia who underwent SERRA DORIA cardioplasty and found that only 38.4% of the patients had normal swallowing and 53.8% of them had regurgitation, concluding that this procedure should only be indicated for patients without clinical conditions justifying esophagectomy.

Based on these considerations, the almost total resection of the esophagus began to acquire a new perspective for the treatment of major achalasia, Camara-Lopes [26], concerned with the poor results of conservative therapy for cases of advanced achalasia of Chagas disease etiology, introduced in Brazil in 1958, the subtotal resection of the esophagus via the right transpleural approach. At the same time, he further recommended that the reconstruction of the transit would be performed in a second surgical stage, through a retrosternal gastroplasty, a surgery that became known after his name.

With the best standardization of this procedure, it was recommended that this surgery be performed at the same time, with the gastric transposition to the cervical region performed by the posterior transmediastinal route, demonstrating the advantages of this technical variant over the previous one, mainly because it leaves the stomach in the space previously occupied by the esophagus, preventing the angulation of the esophagogastric anastomosis; in addition two operative times are avoided, which could cause greater morbidity [27–29].

Although the subtotal esophagus resection could offer the advantage of trying to completely resolve the dysphagia, by removing the entire denervated area of the organ, with great ectasia, it still caused high morbidity [28–30].

Thus, many authors began to indicate more economical resections, acting exclusively in the esophagus distal third section and in the cardia, locations of greatest importance within the achalasia pathophysiology, due to the evident lack of relaxation at the level of the lower esophageal sphincter. Hence, they recommended the distal resection of the organ or simple cardiectomy, either by left thoraco-laparotomy, or laparotomy, reconstructing the transit, either by interposition of a jejunal loop [31–33], or with a colon segment [33, 34] or by means of a valved or non-valved intrathoracic esophagogastric anastomosis [33, 35]. However, mid- and long-term postoperative evaluation with distal esophageal resection showed relapse of dysphagia or gastroesophageal reflux in a significant percentage [31, 32, 34].

Thus, the evaluation, carried out both in anatomical and functional studies, demonstrated with more precision that subtotal esophagectomy was the procedure that was even better suited for the treatment of advanced forms of megaesophagus, despite the great extension of the surgery [36, 37]. In turn, patients with advanced disease, usually malnourished and with difficulty in emptying the esophagus, were predisposed to repeated bronchoaspirations, and may present a significant degree of pulmonary impairment, which causes the transpleural pathway to be predisposed to severe postoperative complications, especially in the pulmonary functions [30, 32, 38].

In the past, the persistence of great surgeons in trying to solve the problem of pulmonary collapse and pleuromediastinal contamination in cases of esophageal cancer led to the recommendation of successful esophagectomy via the cervicoabdominal extrapleural route, in experimental and clinical studies [39].

Based on this experience and always concerned with the obstacle of thoracotomy, over the years, several authors began to indicate esophagectomy without thoracotomy in a rationalized way, in patients with esophagus, cardia or pharyngoesophageal transition malignancy, or even in the case of esophageal stricture, consequence of caustic esophagitis or gastroesophageal reflux [40–44].

Considering that the results were quite favorable, the possibility of performing it for cases of advanced megaesophagus began to be considered. Ferreira [45], seeking to adapt the advantages of subtotal esophagectomy, through a less traumatic technique, especially for patients with severe esophageal ectasia, potentially malnourished and sometimes with pulmonary affections introduced in Brazil cervicoabdominal esophagectomy without thoracotomy, the phleboextraction method, with transit reconstruction through an esophagogastroplasty through the posterior mediastinum, a technique that became known after its author's name.

Thus, with the better standardization of this surgical technique, several authors from the Brazilian surgical school started to use this procedure as a routine in the treatment of advanced megaesophagus [46–49]. Others advocated the resection of the esophagus through the same route, but by rhombodigital mediastinal dissection and detachment [44, 50].

Pinotti [41] and Pinotti et al. [51], improving the evaluation of both procedures, emphasized that they did not provide an adequate approach of the esophagus, and its resection was carried out practically "blindly". Thus, also wanting to avoid the obstacle of thoracotomy, but to provide a wide view of the organ at the mediastinal level for its resection, he proposed a wide frenotomy in the middle portion of the diaphragm, from the esophageal hiatus to the xiphoid appendix. Thus, for more advanced cases of achalasia, a more rationalized technique through the cervicoabdominal approach was deemed suitable. From then on, this technique became known after the name of the author, and was used by other surgeons [49, 50, 52–54].

More recently, with the advent of minimally invasive surgery, resection of the esophagus has been made possible using video laparoscopy [55–57].

Although the resection of the esophagus without thoracotomy, using any of the three technical variations mentioned, could bring the advantages of avoiding the impairment of pulmonary dynamics, such surgery has not been shown to be completely free from complications. Among these, there is the opening of the pleura and consequent hemo or hydropneumothorax, causing greater postoperative morbidity [46, 50, 51, 53, 58]. This can occur, as advanced esophageal achalasia, due to periesophagitis, causes the esophagus to be adhered to the noble structures of the mediastinum and thus during the dissection procedures it may predispose to lesions.

In addition, it is well known that in advanced megaesophagus, stasis esophagitis, which is usually present, predisposes to the development of preneoplastic lesions, such as leukoplakia, and may even progress to malignancy [3, 4, 23, 59, 60].

In view of these considerations, a method was devised that would allow the removal of the esophagus mucosa and submucosa through the esophagus complete invagination, through the combined cervicoabdominal route without thoracotomy and preserving the entire esophageal muscle tunic. Thus, prophylaxis will be performed with the eradication of preneoplastic mucosal lesions that might exist. In addition dissection and detachment of the esophagus at the level of the mediastinum is avoided.

3. Esophageal mucosectomy - historical aspects and indications

The idea of removing the esophageal mucosa and submucosa by invagination, preserving the tunica muscle at the mediastinal level, dates back to 1914 with the pioneering works of Rehn (apud Kirschner [61]). This author, concerned at the time with mediastinal hemorrhages and pleural lesions which occurred in the case of esophageal stripping via the cervical abdominal route in experimental surgery in dogs, conceived the experimental model by extracting only the mucosal and submucosal cylinders through the same route. However, due to the low impact of his method and for not being able to standardize an adequate reconstruction of the cervical esophagus with the stomach, he abandoned his propositions.

Later, other authors demonstrated, in clinical experience, the validity of this procedure in patients with caustic esophagitis, carcinoma of the distal esophagus and of the proximal portion of the stomach [62, 63].

As Brazil is a country with a high incidence of achalasia, mainly due to Chagas etiology, Aquino et al. [64] recommended this type of procedure, initially carrying out an experimental study in dogs, demonstrating its feasibility. Further studies on human cadavers demonstrated the feasibility of this method.

Thus, supported by this experimental verification, our clinical experience began with good evolution in the initial evaluation [65], and recently the great validity of this procedure was demonstrated in 131 patients with advanced achalasia with esophageal diameter greater than 10 cm.

4. Methods – surgical technique: esophageal mucosectomy

Surgical technique following standardization proposed by Aquino [65]:

a. Mucosal resection - Abdominal stage: The surgery starts with a midline laparotomy from the xiphoid process to 5 cm below the umbilicus followed by dissection of the abdominal esophagus and division of vagi nerves. Longitudinal myotomy in the anterior esophagus from the cardia to the hiatus and circumferential dissection of the mucosa/submucosa layer in 5 to 7 cm (**Figure 1**).

   Cervical stage: Left lateral cervicotomy following the anterior border of the sternocleidomastoid muscle from the sternum to 10 cm upwards. Dissection of the esophagus free of the posterior and prevertebral fascia and trachea. Longitudinal myotomy in the anterior esophagus 5 cm from the pharynx to the sternum and circunferencial dissection of the mucosa/submucosa layer. (**Figure 2**).

   Combined stage: After a cylindrical segment of mucosa is dissected free of the muscular in the abdomen and neck, a small mucosectomy is made in the abdomen and neck to allow the passage of a rectal tube upwards. Cervical esophageal mucosa is circumferentially transected and tied to the rectal tube by a long and resistant surgical thread to allow pulling the replacement viscera to the neck. The mucosa is slowly striped downwards and inverted in the abdomen. (**Figures 3** and **4**). The esophagus is completely sectioned at the level of the esophagogastric junction and the neck.

b. Digestive Tract Reconstruction: Digestive tract was reconstructed in all patients with the stomach after division of the left side gastric, right gastroeplicoic and

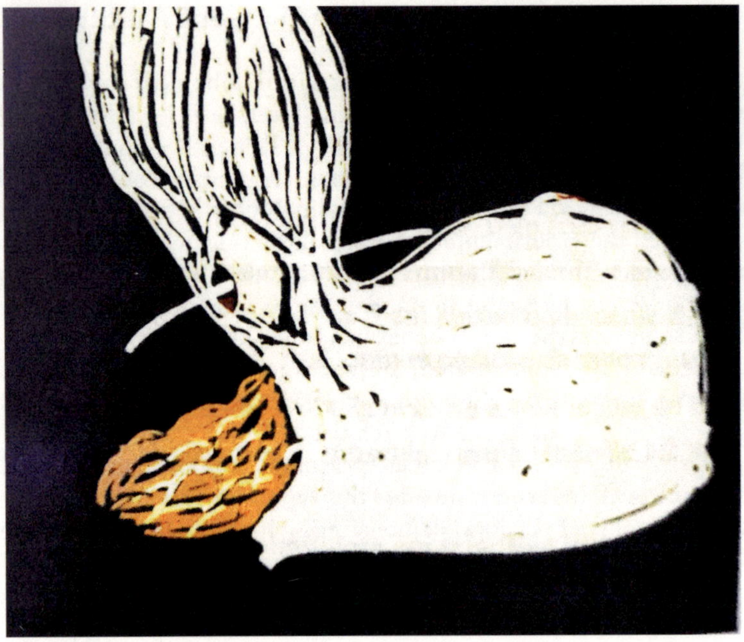

Figure 1.
Abdominal stage-circunferencial dissection of the mucosa/submucosa layer.

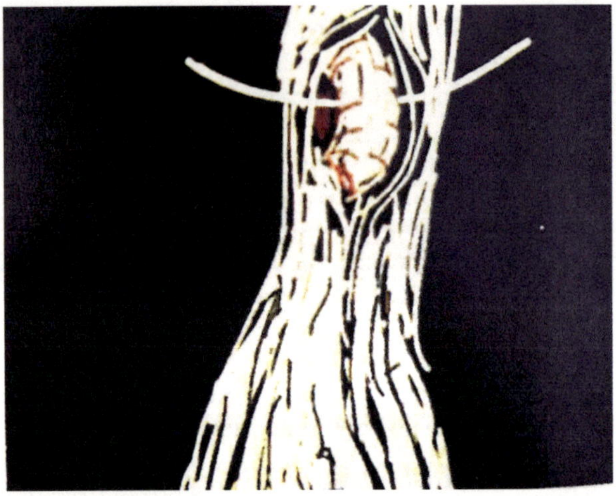

Figure 2.
Cervical stage-circunferencial dissection of the mucosa/submucosa layer.

short vessels. A route for stomach transposition on accessibility to the neck in all patients was into the muscular tunnel (**Figure 5**). Esophagogastrostomy anastomosis was performed at the cervical level too in all patients with a circular stapler for end-to-side anastomosis. A feeding jejunostomy tube was always added to the procedure. Drains were left in the abdomen and neck.

4.1 Early postoperative evaluation

This assessment was performed with 131 patients with advanced achalasia undergoing this type of surgical procedure. The patients remained in the first

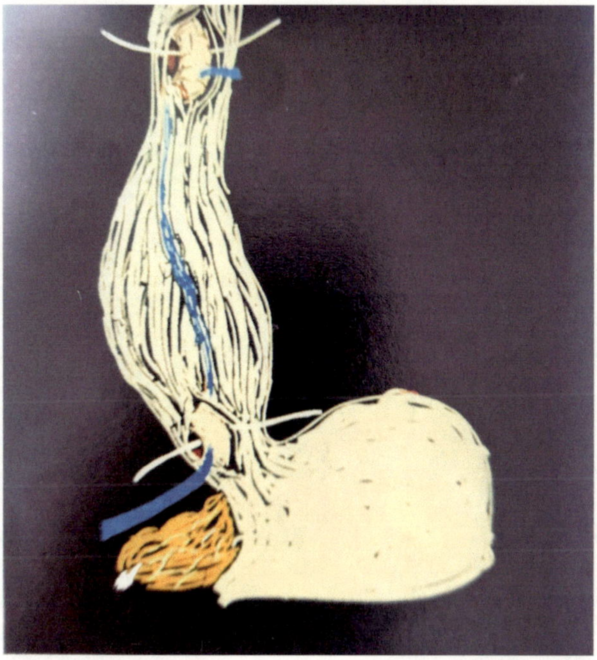

Figure 3.
Cervical esophageal mucosa is transected and tied.

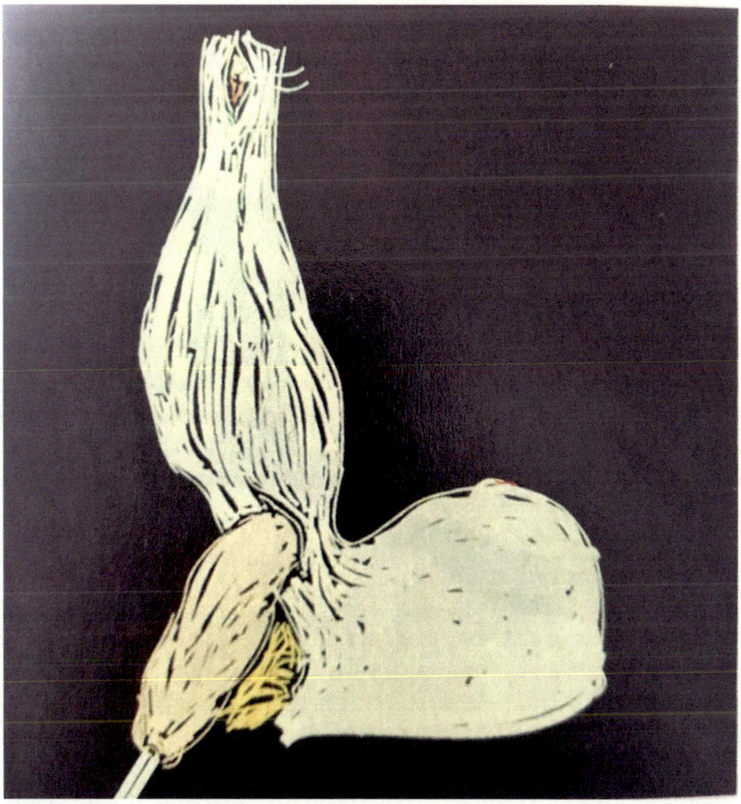

Figure 4.
The mucosa is slowly stripped downwards and inverted in the abdomen.

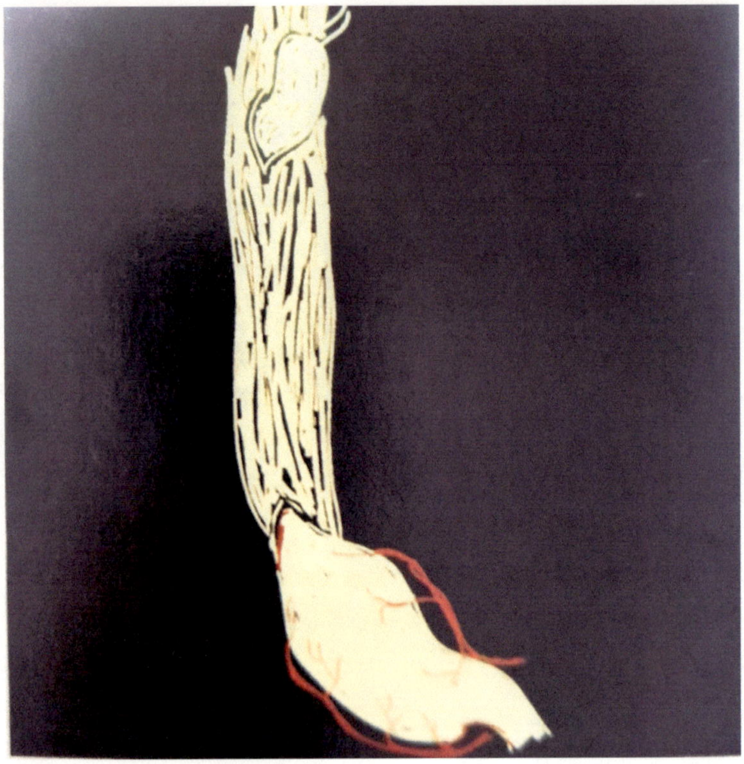

Figure 5.
Gastric transpositon to the neck into the muscular tunnel.

24–48 hours after surgery under the care of the medical team of the Intensive Care Unit, and enteral nutrition was started through the jejunostomy tube, with the reestablishment of intestinal motility.

Oral feedback was instituted after evaluating the integrity of the esophagogastric anastomosis by performing contrast radiography with iodinated substance between the seventh and the tenth postoperative day; in patients with clinical evidence of fistula, depending on its evolution; the day of this examination was variable.

In all patients, a simple chest X-ray was performed in the first 24 hours after surgery and systematically repeated at a 72-hour interval in the first week, or for a shorter period in cases with clinical parameters of pleuropulmonary complications.

The entire sample was initially assessed in terms of morbidity and mortality in the first thirty days after surgery, as well as the treatment for each of the complications.

4.2 Late postoperative evaluation

This assessment was carried out in 85 patients with a variable period of 2 to 5 years after the surgery, and was compared with the preoperative period. The four main clinical symptoms and their intensity was quantified according to the score proposed by Eckardt et al. [66]: (a) DYSPHAGIA: zero - no symptoms; 1- occasional; 2 - daily; 3 - every meal; (b) REGUGITATION: zero - no symptoms; 1- occasional; 2- daily; 3 - every meal; (c) RETROSTERNAL PAIN: zero - no symptoms; 1 - occasional; 2 - daily; 3 - several times a day; WEIGHT LOSS: zero - no loss; 1- <5 kg; 2–5 to 10 kg; 3- > 10 kg.

5. Results

5.1 Early assessment

1. Aspects related to mucosal resection: Mucosal resection by means of submucosal detachment was performed easily and without accidents in all 131 patients, with the removal of the entire circumference of that tunic.

2. Anatomopathological evaluation: In all surgical samples studied, there was moderate to intense lymphoplasmacytic infiltrate, both in the mucosal and submucosal layers. In 17 surgical specimens (12.9%), leukoplastic lesions were present, but none of them showed malignancy.

3. Clinical evaluation: out of the 131 patients studied, 129 (98.4%) had good evolution without any hemodynamic changes, being discharged from the Intensive Care Unit within the first 48 hours after surgery. Oral diet started between the 7th and 10th postoperative day in 107 patients (83.0%), after confirmation of the integrity of the cervical esophagogastric anastomosis by the esophagram. The jejunostomy tube was removed after 3 to 4 weeks postoperatively when solid diet was introduced orally. In 22 patients (17.0%), due to anastomotic dehiscence, the oral diet was reintroduced between the 18th and 29th day after surgery, after clinical and radiological confirmation of the closure of the anastomotic dehiscence.

4. Chest radiological evaluation: Simple chest radiography performed postoperatively on the recommended days did not reveal any pleuropulmonary alteration in 113 patients (86.2%). In the remaining ones, isolated pleural effusion was evidenced in 11 patients (8.3%), pulmonary infiltrate only in 5 patients (3.8%) and association of pleural effusion and pulmonary infiltrate in 2 patients (1.5%).

5. Complications – Two patients (1.5%) died on the third and fifth postoperative days, for sepsis due to stomach necrosis and pulmonary embolism, respectively. Chest drainage was performed in 7 of the 11 patients who presented with moderate pleural effusion, with expectant management for the remaining 4 patients and with good outcome. Pulmonary infection diagnosed in 7 patients (7.6%) was treated with specific medication and with good evolution. Anastomotic dehiscence present in 22 patients had good resolution with conservative treatment. Of these, 9 patients had anastomotic stenosis, with good improvement after endoscopic dilation.

Symptoms	N = 85 patients		
	Preoperative	Postoperative (2 to 5 years)	*p*
Dysphagia	2.7	0.9	<0.001
Regurgitation	2.1	0.8	0.043
Retrosternal pain	1.9	0.2	0.049
Weight loss	2.9	0.0	0.001
Total	9.6	1.9	0.009

Table 1.
Distribution of patients in the pre- and postoperative period in relation to the mean of symptoms according to the Eckardt score et al. [66].

5.2 Late assessment

It was performed in 85 patients between 2 and 5 years after the surgery in relation to the average of the four symptoms recommended by the Ekardt et al. score [66], A significant difference between the pre- and postoperative periods was observed during the time studied, showing that the patients experienced a good evolution (**Table 1**). And also when taking the mean of the sum of symptoms, the difference was also very significant, because preoperatively the mean score was 9.6 and postoperatively it decreased to 1.9 (**Table 1**).

6. Comments

Most of the time, the few authors who described the clinical experience of removal of the mucosa and submucosa of the esophagus by invagination with preservation of the muscular tunic performed median frenotomy with section of the diaphragmatic pillar for greater exposure of the esophagus, and thus to be able to dissect the mucosa in greater detail extension [62, 63].

Opening the diaphragm with greater esophageal dissection at the mediastinal level would not correspond to one of the objectives recommended by the technique we propose: to avoid mediastinal involvement. Thus, in no patient in the series studied, this exposure became necessary, since the dissection of the mucosa in relation to the tunica muscularis, performed along the entire length of the abdominal esophagus and in almost the entire length of the cervical esophagus, was sufficient for the removal of the specimen with the surgical procedure in all the cases studied, according to intraoperative macroscopic evaluation.

This easy removal of the mucosa through the submucosal plane must occur due to the histological characteristics of the esophagus tunics. The mucosa consists of a resistant stratified flat epithelium, and the submucosa has a low proportion of collagen fibers and a large amount of elastic fibers, making it more flexible and looser [62].

Another objective of this procedure is that in the entire resection of the mucosal/submucosal cylinder, both the prophylaxis and the eradication of all chronic inflammatory lesions detected due to the long-term food stasis and, as a consequence, a malignant potential, have occurred as has been shown in some series of patients with advanced megaesophagus, with a frequency ranging from 3–10% [3, 27, 49, 50]. The presence of carcinoma was not found in any of the samples, although in all cases, there was moderate to intense inflammatory infiltrate and in 12.9% leukoplastic lesions.

Mediastinal hemorrhage is not a common occurrence after esophagectomy without thoracotomy. However, a high incidence of morbidity and mortality is expected when hemorrhage occurs [29, 33, 42, 44]. This can occur due to direct injury to the azygos vein and esophageal vessels directly from the aorta, which associated with pleural involvement can progress to hemothorax in up to 25% of cases. This complication usually requires immediate repair by thoracotomy, often unsuccessfully, a fact that did not occur in any of the cases of esophageal mucosectomy technique surgeries used.

Another complication that can occur with transhiatal esophagectomy is hydropneumothorax with an index variable from 22.2% to 83.3%, because the dissection of the esophagus at the mediastinal level can result in the opening of the pleura [29, 33, 42, 44–46]. The reduced incidence of pleuropulmonary complications and none at the mediastinal level in the series of patients in our study, justifies once again the proposed technical procedure.

Recently, Aquino et al. [67] compared intra- and postoperative complications in 229 patients with advanced megaesophagus undergoing esophageal mucosectomy and transhiatal esophagectomy. Pleural effusion with or without hemothorax was more frequent in patients submitted to transhiatal. Other complications of great morbidity occurred only in the group submitted to transhiatal, like massive hemothorax which developed in 6 (5%) patients, among which two died. Also in the transhiatal groups, 3 (2%) patients developed tracheal injury and one of them died.

Another important aspect to consider with this technique is the possibility of excessive bleeding when removing the mucosa and submucosa. However, both in the intra- and immediate postoperative evaluation, all parameters showed that the patients evolved hemodynamically stable and few required blood replacement. Paricio et al. [62] demonstrated in their series that the amount of blood did not exceed 100 mL by aspiration drainage from the tunica muscularis in 3 patients who had undergone mucosectomy due to adenocarcinoma of the cardia. Other authors who also performed this technique demonstrated that although the mean blood volume eliminated intraoperatively was between 700 to 800 mL, in none of the patients hemodynamic instability developed [63]. Aquino et al. [64], demonstrated in an experimental study in dogs, absence of active bleeding 2 hours after mucosectomy.

These findings confirming the minor bleeding with the use of the technique described above may be due to the characteristics of the esophagus intramural blood supply. According to Potter & Holyoke [68], the segmental arterial branches of the aorta penetrate the longitudinal and circular muscle bundles of the esophageal wall and further subdivide into the highly distensible tunica submucosa. Thus since these vessels have a much narrower caliber than the esophagus arteries it is supposed that spontaneous hemostasis occurs.

In the late evaluation of the 85 patients whom we were able to follow-up up for 5 years, the validity of said operative procedure was evidenced once again, because, as demonstrated, the four symptoms recommended by Eckardt et al. score [66] had an evident significance between the pre- and post-operative period with good evolution of the patients. Dysphagia stands out, which in the preoperative period all patients exhibited this symptom daily and/or at every meal and in the postoperative period, the majority had normal swallowing or very occasional dysphagia. In addition, all patients experienced a very expressive weight gain with 27 patients exhibiting more than 25 kg of weight gain.

And also when we evaluated the mean sum of symptoms at the same time of follow-up, the good evolution of the patients was once again confirmed, as preoperatively it was 9.6 and post-operatively it decreased significantly to 1.9.

Until the presentation of our study, no series had demonstrated any study that could compare in the preoperative and postoperative esophagectomy period performed for advanced achalasia of chagasic or idiopathic origin, the assessment of the sum of the symptom score proposed by Eckardt et al. [66]. Only this author's study is reported with 54 patients with idiopathic achalasia, but who underwent pneumatic dilation with a mean follow-up of 13.8 years after the procedure. These authors recommended that in order to have clinical remission of the disease after treatment, it is necessary that the symptoms have completely disappeared or that the total sum of the score does not exceed 3, a fact that was very evident in our series.

Thus, we conclude that esophageal mucosectomy with preservation of the muscular tunic for the treatment of advanced esophageal achalasia is an adequate procedure due to the low incidence of pleuropulmonary complications, absence of mediastinal complications and good resolution of symptoms in the long term. We thus hope to offer a new alternative for those who consider the esophagus resectability as the best form of therapy for advanced achalasia.

Acknowledgements

To Hospital Puc-Campinas.

Conflict of interest

The authors declare no conflict of interest.

Author details

José Luis Braga de Aquino* and Vânia Aparecida Leandro-Merhi
Postgraduate Program of Health Sciences, Pontifical Catholic University of Campinas, Campinas, SP, Brazil

*Address all correspondence to: jlaquino@sigmanet.com.br

References

[1] Aquino JLB, Said MM, Camargo JGT. Non-conventional surgical approach to achalasia: mucosectomy and endomuscular pull-through. Mini-invasive Surg. 2017;1:167-172.

[2] Zaninotto G, Bennet C, Boeckxstaens G, Costatini M, Ferguson MK, Pandolfino JE, et al. The 2018 ISDE achalasia guidelines. Dis Esophagus. 2018;31(9):1-29. DOI: 10.1093/dote/doy071. PMID: 30169645.

[3] Vaezi MF, Pandolfino JE, Yadiapati RH, Greer KB, Kavit RT. ACG Clinical Guidelines: diagnosis and management of achalasia. Am J Gastroenterol. 2020;115:1393-1411.

[4] Jung HK, Hong SJ, Lee OY, Pandolfino JE, Park H, MiwaH, et al. 2019 Seoul Consensus on Esophageal Achalasia Guidelines. J Neurogastroenterol Motil. 2020;26(2):180-203.

[5] Rezende JM. Historia da cirurgia da acalasia do esôfago e do megaesôfago chagásico. 4ª ed. Goiânia: Editora Kelps; 2011 [citado 20 nov. 2017]. Disponível em: http://www.jmrezende.com.br/acalasia.htm. Portuguese.

[6] Andreollo NA, Earlam RJ. Heller's myotomy for achalasia: is an added anti-reflux procedure necessary? Br J Surg. 1987;74(9):765-769.

[7] Donahue PE, Schlesinger PK, Sluss KF, Richter HM, Liu KJ, Nyhus LM. Esophagocardiomyotomy floppy Nissen fundoplication effectively treats achalasia without causin gesophageal obstruction. Surgical. 1994;116(4):719-725.

[8] Andolfi C, Fisichella PM. Meta-analysis of clinical outcome after treatment for achalasia based on manometric subtypes. Br J Surg. 2019;106(4):332-341.

[9] Campos GM, Vittinghoff E, Rabl C. Endoscopic and surgical treatments for achalasia: A systematic review and meta-analysis. Ann Surg. 2009;249(1):45-57.

[10] Ramchandani M, Nageshwar DR, NabiZ. Management of achalasia cardia: expert consensus statements. J Gastroenterol Hepatol. 2018;33(8):1436-1444.

[11] Inoue H, Minami H, Kobayashi Y. Per oral endoscopic myotomy (POEM) for esophageal achalasia. Endoscopy. 2010;42(4):265-271.

[12] Ponds FA, Fockens P, Lei A. Effect of peroral endoscopic myotomy vs pneumatic dilation on symptom severity and treatment outcomes among treatment-naive patients with achalasia: a randomized clinical trial. JAMA. 2019;322(2):134-144.

[13] Park CH, Jung DH, Kim DH. Comparative efficacy of per-oral endoscopic myotomy and heller myotomy in patiens with achalasia: a meta-analysis. Gastrointest Endosc. 2019;90:546-558.

[14] Peng L, Tian S, Du C, Yuan Z,GuoM, Lu L. Outcome of per-oral endoscopic myotomy (POEM) for treating achalasia compared with laparoscopic heller myotomy (LHM). Surg Laparosc Endosc Percutan Tech. 2017;27:60-64.

[15] De Pascale S, Repici A, Puccetti F, Carlani E, Rosati R, Fumagalli U. Per oral endoscopic myotomy versus surgical myotomy for primary achalasia: single-center, retrospectiveanalysis of 74 patients. Dis Esophagus. 2017;30:1-7.

[16] Li QL, Wu QN, Zhang XC. Outcomes of per-oral endoscopic myotomy for treatment of esophageal achalasia with a median follow-up of 49 months. Gastrointest Endosc. 2018;87:1405-1412.

[17] Repeci A, Fuccio L, Maselli R. GERD afterper-oral endoscopic myotomy as compared with Heller's myotomy with fundoplication: a systematic review with meta-analysis. Gastrointest Endosc. 2018;87(4):934-943.

[18] Schottmann F, Luckett DJ, Fine J. Laparoscopic Heller myotomy versus peroralendoscopicmyoomy (POEM) for achalasia: a systematic review and meta-analysis. Ann Surg. 2018;267(3):451-460.

[19] Brandalise NA, Leonardi LS, Mantovani M, Fagundes JJ. Tratamento cirúrgico do megaesofago: estudo comparativo entre duas técnicas de cardioplastia. Rev Col Bras Cir. 1979;6(3);117-120. Portuguese.

[20] Malafaia O, Brenner S, Costa e Silva IT, Guelfi SB, Bacelar MCL, Artigas GV. Tratamento cirúrgico do megaesôfago pela técnica de Thal. Rev Col Bras Cir. 1981;8(3):111-118. Portuguese.

[21] Serra Doria OB, Serra Doria OM, Serra Doria OR, Doria JC. Operação de Serra-Doria para o tratamento do megaesôfago: considerações quanto a originalidade do método. Ann Paul Med Cir. 1972;99(2):113-120. Portuguese.

[22] Nakadaira AA, Benedicto JM, Galletti H, Silva Filho AF, Pinotti HW. Tratamento do megaesôfago pela técnica de Thal. Rev Assoc Med Bras. 1974;20(10):371-373. Portuguese.

[23] Ximenes Netto M, Marra O, Debiase H, Gomide JC, França AT, Silva RO. Primary surgical treatment of Chagas' megaesophagus: results of 450 cases. HFA Publ Tec Cient 1987;2(2):147-161.

[24] Ponciano H, Ceconello I, Alves L, Ferreira BD, Gama-Rodrigues JJ. Cardioplasty and Roux in Y parcial gastrectomy (Serra Doria procedure) for reoperation of achalasia. Arq Gastroenterol. 2004;41:155-161.

[25] Aquino JLB, Said MM, Pereira DAR, Leandro-Merhi VA, Nascimento PC, Reis VV. Early and late assessment of esophagocardioplasty in the surgical treatment of advanced recurrent megaesophagus. Arq Gastroenterol. 2016;53:53:235-239.

[26] Camara-Lopes LH. Esofagoplastia com estomago por tunelização retrosternal. Rev Paul Med. 1958;53:149-153. Portuguese.

[27] Camara-Lopes LH, Ferreira-Santos R. Indicação seletiva do processo de Heller, da ressecção parcial e da ressecção subtotal do esôfago no tratamento cirúrgico do megaesôfago: analise critica da experiência do Departamento de Cirurgia da Faculdade de Medicina de Ribeirão Preto. Rev Paul Med. 1958;52:269-275. Portuguese.

[28] Azevedo PC, Sequeira OF, Santos EM, Pimentel Netto O, França GE. Tratamento cirúrgico de afecções do esôfago pela técnica de Camara Lopes. Rev Bras Cir. 1963;46:2-19. Portuguese.

[29] Orringer MB, Stirling MC. Esophageal resection for achalasia: indications and results. Ann Thorac Surg. 1989;47:340-345.

[30] RassiL. Critério seletivo na indicação da técnica cirúrgica para o megaesôfago chagásico. Rev Goiana Med. 1979;25:85-104. Portuguese.

[31] Resende JS. Tratamento cirúrgico do megaesôfago- operação de Merendino. Rev Goiana Med. 1973;19(3/4):169-184. Portuguese.

[32] Lazáro da Silva A, Conceição SA, Silva MLA. Interposição de alça jejunal no tratamento cirúrgico do megaesôfago chagásico: analise do pós-operatório imediato. Rev Assoc Med Bras. 1987;33(5/6):94-98. Portuguese.

[33] Moreno Gonzales E, Garcia Alvarez A, Landa Garcia I, Gomez Gutierrez M, Rico Selas P, Garcia Garcia JI. Results of surgical treatment of esophageal achalasia. Multicenter retrospective study of 1856 cases. Int Surg. 1988;73:69-77.

[34] Barbosa H, Barichello AW, Vianna AL, Mendelssonh P, Wata-NabeLM. Tratamento cirúrgico do megaesôfago chagásico: duas décadas de experiência numa região endêmica. Rev Goiana Med. 1989;35:1-23. Portuguese.

[35] Ellis JR FH, CrozierRE, GibbSP. Reoperative achalasia surgery. J Thorac Cardiovasc Surg. 1986;92(5);859-865.

[36] Koberle F. Patogênese dos megas. Rev Goiana Med. 1956;2(2):101-110. Portuguese.

[37] Godoy RA. Estudo da esofagopatia chagásica crônica por meio do método eletromanométrico e da prova da metacolina em pacientes com e sem dilatação do esôfago. Rev Goiana Med. 1972;18(112):1-73. Portuguese.

[38] Santos MIR, Guida Filho B. Resultados do tratamento cirúrgico do megaesôfago no paciente tuberculoso. Rev Paul Med. 1969;75-105-112. Portuguese.

[39] Turner GG. Carcinoma of the oesophagus: the question of its treatment by surgery. Lancet. 1936;1:130-134.

[40] Le Quesne LP, Ranger D. Pharyngolaryngectomy with immediate pharyngo gastric anastomosis. Br J Surg. 1966;53(2):105-109.

[41] Pinotti HW. Esofagectomia subtotal por túnel transmediastinal sem toracotomia. Ver Assoc Med Bras. 1977;23(11):395-398. Portuguese.

[42] Moreno Gonzalez E, Hidalgo Pascual M, Moreno Azcoita M, Garcia Garcia JI, Garcia Blanch G, Rico Selas P. Indicaciones, técnica y resultados de la esofaguectomia transhiatal digital sin toracotomia. Rev Esp Enferm Apar Dig. 1981;60(6):533-558. Spanish.

[43] Orringer MB, Sloan H. Esophagectomy without thoracotomy. J Thorac Cardiovasc Surg. 1978;76(5):643-654.

[44] Orringer MB. Transhiatal esophagectomy for benign disease. J Thorac Cardiovasc Surg. 1985;90(5):649-655.

[45] Ferreira EAB. Esofagectomia subtotal, pro via cervicoabdominal combinada: sua possível utilização no megaesôfago. Rev Paul Med. 1973; 82(3/4):133-134. Portuguese.

[46] Pareja JC, Lacerda JC, Amorim Filho J, Paranagua DF, Fonseca PC. O tratamento cirúrgico do megaesôfago grau IV pela técnica de Ferreira: esofagectomia subtotal e esofagogastroplastia transmediastinal posterior sem toracotomia. Rev Assoc Med Bras. 1978;24(2):66-68. Portuguese.

[47] Ferraz EM, Bacelar TS, Lacerda CM, Lima FEA, Souza AP, KelnerS. Tratamento cirúrgico do megaesôfago chagásico: avaliação de 60 casos. An Paul Med Cir. 1981;108(4):9-18. Portuguese.

[48] Cunha ASB. Esofagectomia subtotal com anastomose esofagogástrica cervical transmediastinal sem toracotomia para tratamento do megaesôfago. Rev Col Bras Cir. 1981;8(4);159-160. Portuguese.

[49] Ximenes Netto M. Megaesophagus: current review of techniques and results. Rev Saúde. 1991;2(4):207-236.

[50] ORRINGER MB, STIRLING MC. Esophageal resection for achalasia: indications and results. Ann Thorac Surg. 1989;47:340-345.

[51] Pinotti HW, Pollara WM, Raia AA. Tratamento cirúrgico do megaesôfago avançado pela esofagectomia subtotal por via cervico abdominal sem toracotomia com abertura do diafragma. Rev Assoc Med Bras. 1980;26(10):339-342. Portuguese.

[52] Cecconello I, Domene CE, Sallum RAA, Pinotti HW. Esofagectomia transmediastinal no megaesôfago. Rev Col Bras Cir. 1988;15:76-81. Portuguese.

[53] Andreollo NA, Brandalise NA, Lopes LR, Leonardi LS, Pantoja M. A esofagectomia sem toracotomia no tratamento do megaesôfago chagásico avançado. Rev Col Bras Cir. 1988;15:43-47. Portuguese.

[54] Sabas AA, Abdala JE. Esofagectomia total sin toracotomia en acalasia. Rev Fac Cienc Med Univ Nac Cuyo. 1984;7(1):26-27. Spanish.

[55] Crema E, Ribeiro LBP, Souza RC, Terra Junior JÁ, Silva BF, Silva AA. Esofagectomia transhiatal laparoscopica para o tratamento do megaesôfago avançado: Analise de 60 casos. Rev Col Bras Cir. 2009;36(2):118-122. Portuguese.

[56] Smithers BM, Gotley DC, Martin JM. Comparison of the outcomes between open and minimally invasive esophagectomy. Ann Surg. 2007;24(2):232-40.

[57] Fontan AJA, Batista Neto J, Pontes ACP, Nepomuceno MC, Muritiba TG, Furtado RS. Minimally invasive laparoscopic esophagectomy vs transhiatal open esophagectomy in achalasia: a randomized study. ABCD Arq Bras Cir Dig. 2018;31(3):24-29.

[58] Orringer MB, Marshall B, Stirling MC. Transhiatal esophagectomy for benign and malignant disease. J Thorac Cardiovasc Surg. 1993; 105(2):265-277.

[59] Brandalise NA, Andreollo NA, Leonardi LS, Callejas NETO F. Carcinoma associado ao megaesôfago chagásico. Rev Col Bras Cir. 1985;12(6):196-199. Portuguese.

[60] Goodman P, Scott LD, Verani RR, Berggeen CC. Esophageal adenocarcinoma in a patient with surgically treated achalasia. Dig Dis Sci. 1990;35(12):1549-1552.

[61] Kirschner M. Operaciones en la cavidad toracica. Intervenciones en el carcinoma del esôfago. In: Tratado de técnica operatória general e y especial. Barcelona: Editorial Labor; 1944. Parte 2:985-1020. Spanish.

[62] Parrilla Paricio P, Aguayo Albasini JL, Ponce Marco JL. "Stripping" esofágico submucoso com técnica de esofagectomia sin toracotomia: estudo clinico y experimental. Cir Esp. 1984;38:546-552. Spanish.

[63] Saidi F, Abbassi A, Shadmehr MB, Khoshnevis-ASL G. Endothoracic endoesophageal pull-trough operation: a new approach to cancers of the esophagus and proximal stomach. J Thoracic Cardiovasc Surg. 1991;102 (1):43-50.

[64] Aquino JLB, Moraes SP, Martinez SE, Said MM, Reis Neto JA. Esofagectomia submucosa. Acta Cir Bras. 1989;4(1);64-65. Portuguese.

[65] Aquino JLB. Tratamento do megaesôfago pela mucosectomia com conservação da túnica muscular esofágica por via cervicoabdominal [tese]. Campinas: Universidade Estadual de Campinas; 1996. Portuguese.

[66] Eckardt VF, Gockel I, Bernhard G. Pneumatic dilation to achalasia: late results of a prospective follow-up in investigation. Gut. 2004;53:629-633.

[67] Aquino JLB, Said MM, Pereira DAR, Machado FR, Ramos JPZ,

Brandi LA, et al. Análise comparativa da mucosectomia esofágica e da esofagectomia transmediastinal no tratamento do megaesôfago avançado: estudo comparativo em 229 pacientes [Português]. In: Anais do XXXII Congresso Brasileiro de Cirurgia, 2017, São Paulo. São Paulo: CBC; 2017. Portuguese.

[68] Potter SE, Holyoke EA. Observations on the intrinsic blood supply of the esophagus. Arch Surg. 1950;61;944-948.

Chapter 7

Lipofilling in Post-Treatment Oral Dysfunction in Head and Neck Cancer Patients

Marise Neijman, R.T. Karsten, L. van der Molen, O. Lapid and M.W.M. van den Brekel

Abstract

Lipofilling is a new treatment option for head- and neck cancer patients who suffer from chronic and severe (chemo-) radiation or surgery-related swallowing problems. Lipofilling is a technique of autologous grafting in which living fat cells are transplanted from one location to another in the same patient. In the case of head and neck cancer patients, volume loss or muscle atrophy of the tongue or pharyngeal musculature caused by the treatment may result in oropharyngeal dysfunction. Firstly, intensive swallowing therapy will be given, but if that offers no further improvement and the functional problems persist, lipofilling can be considered. By transplantation of autologous adipose tissue, the functional outcomes might improve by compensating the existing tissue defects or tissue loss. Only a few studies have been published which evaluated the effectiveness of this new treatment option. The results of those studies show that the lipofilling technique seems safe and of potential value for improving swallowing function in some of the included patients with chronic and severe dysphagia after surgery and/or (chemo-) radiation therapy for head and neck cancer. The lipofilling procedure will be described in detail as well as the clinical implications.

Keywords: lipofilling, head and neck neoplasms, dysphagia, deglutition, deglutition disorders, fat transfer, autologous fat injection, adipose tissue, quality of life

1. Introduction

Head and Neck Cancer (HNC) is the seventh most common type of cancer worldwide [1]. The regions of HNC include cancers of the nasal cavity, oral cavity, nasopharynx, oropharynx, hypopharynx, larynx, and paranasal sinuses (see **Figure 1**). Risk factors are tobacco use, alcohol consumption [2], and viral infections with the Human Papilloma Virus (HPV) (for oropharyngeal cancers) [3] and Epstein-Barr Virus (EPV) (for nasopharyngeal cancers) [4].

1.1 TNM classification

HNC tumors can be classified using the TNM stage classification published by the American Joint Committee on Cancer and International Union for Cancer

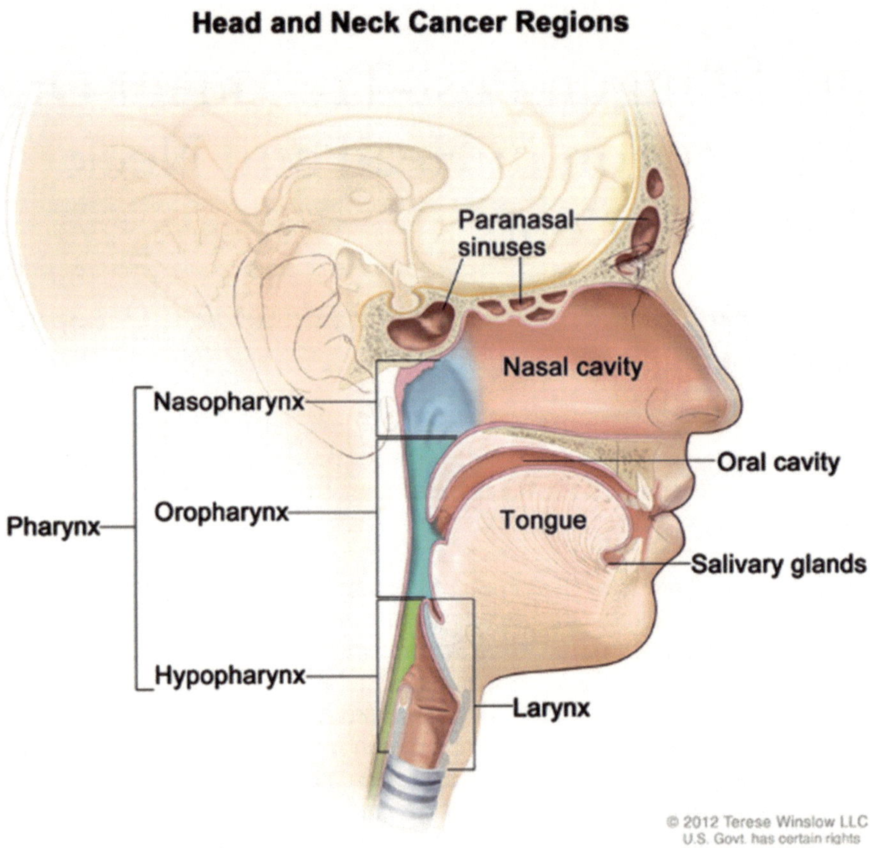

Figure 1.
Regions of head and neck cancer, source: https://www.intechopen.com/chapters/67124

Committee (AJCC/UICC) [5]. This classification is based on the anatomic tumor extent and includes three different aspects. Firstly, the size of the primary tumor (T), secondly the presence or absence and extent of involved regional lymph nodes (N), and lastly the presence or absence of distant metastasis (M). With the TNM classification, it is possible to give an estimate on cancer prognosis and it is helpful for treatment selection and proper communication. An example of a TNM classified advanced oropharynx carcinoma with one lymph node involved and diagnosed with no distant metastasis is T3N1M0.

1.2 Head and neck cancer treatment

Patients with HNC can be treated with (a combination of) surgery, radiotherapy, chemotherapy, proton therapy, immunotherapy, or photodynamic therapy (PDT). The choice of treatment depends on the location and the size of the tumor (TNM classification). Despite improved radiotherapy techniques, the anatomical structures, including muscles and tissue around the primary tumor, can still be damaged by the tumor itself or the treatment [6–8]. Well-known (negative) side effects of the HNC treatment are xerostomia, sticky saliva, mucositis, altered taste, weight loss, pain, trismus and tissue loss due to fibrosis. Long-term functional problems such as swallowing problems (dysphagia), voice or speech problems, and trismus can harm patients' quality of life [9].

2. Dysphagia in HNC patients

One of the most critical and potentially life-threatening functional problems in patients who are treated for advanced HNC is acute and chronic dysphagia. One of the causes of dysphagia after HNC treatment might be a reduced tongue strength, insufficient contact between the base of tongue and pharyngeal wall, reduced hyolaryngeal elevation, and reduced opening of the upper esophageal sphincter. Due to this altered physiology, the food bolus is swallowed less powerfully, leading to stagnation of food ('residue'), with a high risk of laryngeal penetration or even (silent) laryngeal aspiration of the residue into the trachea. The swallowing problems may worsen when the swallowing musculature is no longer actively used, and the so-called 'non-use' atrophy occurs, causing further deterioration of the swallowing function [10]. Dysphagia (chronic) can lead to reduced body weight, long-term and even lifelong feeding tube dependency, depression, reduced quality of life, aspiration pneumonia and can even lead to death [6, 11, 12].

3. Treatment options of HNC related dysphagia

In the next paragraph, the treatment options of HNC-related dysphagia will be described. Firstly, the importance of interdisciplinary head and neck rehabilitation will be described, secondly (preventive) swallowing protocols and finally, surgical options.

3.1 Interdisciplinary head and neck rehabilitation

The treatment of dysphagia, and the treatment of HNC patients in general, involves a high level of variety and complexity of problems. Therefore, it is recommended to have a specialized multidisciplinary team of medical specialists and allied health professionals, specialized in head and neck oncology [13]. Rehabilitative care aims primarily at reducing and/or preventing negative effects of head and neck cancer treatment, and thereby improving daily functioning. The effectiveness of head and neck rehabilitation program have been proven [13, 14].

3.2 (Preventive) swallowing protocols

Over the last years, the prevention of dysphagia has become a major focus point in HNC research. The assumed disadvantages of (prophylactic) feeding tube placement to prevent weight loss and with that effectively immobilizing the swallowing musculature, have led to the so-called 'eat or exercise' principle [10]. This means that oral intake should be maintained as long as possible, and that preventive swallowing rehabilitation programs should keep the swallowing musculature 'active' as much as possible before and during treatment. Studies on preventive rehabilitation in the Netherlands and elsewhere have shown that preventive swallowing protocols (in particular in the short-term) are associated with better post-treatment functional outcomes and quality of life, and are cost-effective, compared to standard care [10, 15–22].

There are several (swallowing) exercises that have proven their value in the treatment of dysphagia. Those exercises are used in standard swallowing protocols, but also within preventive rehabilitation protocols. Most frequently used exercises include a range of motion or resistance exercises (with or without medical devices such as the TheraBite® device), compensatory techniques (postural changes, diet/bolus modifications), behavioral swallow exercises such as the (super-)supraglottic swallow [23, 24], the effortful swallow [25], the Mendelsohn maneuver [26], and the Masako (tongue-holding) maneuver [27], and non-swallow exercises such as the Shaker (head-raising) exercise [28]. Also, devices, such as the Swallow Exercise Aid (SEA) have been developed to be able to perform multiple exercises more efficiently. The SEA device allows adaptation to individual subjects' capacity, and thus the application of progressive overload during the training program, and has shown to activate important swallowing structures [29–31]. Nevertheless, in some cases severe, therapy-refractory dysphagia may still exist.

3.3 Surgical procedures

Surgical treatment of functional impairment may be considered when rehabilitative measures, such as those described above, are insufficient to help ensure safe and efficient oral intake. The primary goals of surgery are to reduce the risk of aspiration, improve bolus transfer, and prevent malnutrition and/or dehydration. What the best surgical technique will depend on the etiology of the dysphagia. If there is less relaxation of the upper esophageal sphincter this can result in a less efficient movement of the bolus into the esophagus. This impaired relaxation can sometimes be remedied by reducing the tonus of the musculature of the pharynx. Cricopharyngeal myotomy, either endoscopically using a CO_2 laser or by an open surgical procedure, can be helpful [32, 33]. Myotomy of the cricopharyngeal muscle results in lower resistance of the upper esophageal sphincter. Due to this lower resistance, the bolus can be more easily be transported through the upper esophageal sphincter and enter the esophagus.

Other surgical techniques that can widen the cricopharyngeal muscle are dilatation (in case of fibrosis) or botulinum toxin (botox) injection in case of spasm. Several studies have reported promising results in patients with upper esophageal sphincter dysfunction caused by muscle spasm or hypertonicity [34, 35].

If dysphagia is caused by a serious limitation in laryngeal elevation, an invasive surgical technique called hyolaryngeal suspension can be performed. In this procedure, the hyoid bone is suspended and the thyroid-cricoid complex is fixated to the anterior mandible. This results in a permanent more cranial position of the larynx [36]. This procedure can be very effective in the restore a full oral intake without aspiration. However, it is also reported that previous treatment with (chemo) radiotherapy will negatively influence the outcome [37].

Finally, in some cases, none of the abovementioned treatment options are suitable or effective. If the larynx has severe functional impairments and there is no reasonable likelihood of functional recovery as a 'last refuge', a functional total laryngectomy can be considered. In the case of a total laryngectomy, the airway is surgically separated from the digestive tract by sacrificing the larynx.

Surgery procedures as described above, however, can have serious complication risks. Myotomy (especially open) can cause infections and even pharyngocutaneous fistulas or (retropharyngeal) infection [34, 37]. Besides, studies have shown that the improvement rate is much higher for neurologic dysphagia and idiopathic dysfunction than in patients with swallowing problems due to HNC treatment [32].

4. New treatment option: lipofilling

Since 2013, the Netherlands Cancer Institute has been using lipofilling as an alternative treatment option. Lipofilling has the advantage of being less radical, less invasive and presenting less of a burden for the patients [38].

Lipofilling is a technique in which autologous fat is transplanted to a site that lacks volume. In 1893, fat was transplanted for the first time with variable success [39]. Since the 1980s with the advent of modern liposuction, the technique of lipofilling has become a standard modality for esthetic as well as reconstructive purposes; however, it is rarely used in HNC patients.

4.1 *Physiology of fat grafting*

Of all tissues in the human body, fat possesses the highest percentage of adipose-derived stem cells with more than 5.000 of these per gram of fat. Adipose-derived stem cells are present in the mesenchyme, and are a type of multipotent stem cells. This means that these stem cells can differentiate into multiple cell types including osteoblasts, endothelial cells, myocytes, neuronal type cells, adipocytes and chondrocytes [40, 41].

A microscopic view shows that fat consists of a complex matrix of adipocytes mixed with collagen, endothelial cells, adipose-derived stem cells, and fibroblasts. All these adipocytes play an important role in the physiological processes, such as angiogenesis, metabolism, lipid storage and endocrine functions [40]. There is evidence that stem cells may even contribute to the reduction in fibrosis, and the restoration of tissue vascularization and organ function [42, 43].

4.2 Evaluation tools to check patient eligibility

Lipofilling might be a suitable treatment option for specific patients with chronic dysphagia after HNC treatment. Patients might benefit from lipofilling when part of the etiology of the dysphagia consists of lack of volume, for instance, of the tongue or pharyngeal wall. There are different examination tools to analyze the severity and etiology of dysphagia. Before considering if lipofilling is suitable for a patient, it is recommended to perform objective assessments such as Fiberoptic Endoscopic Evaluation of Swallowing (FEES) or a Video Fluoroscopic Swallow Study (VFSS) and a Magnetic Resonance Imaging (MRI) assessment.

FEES, in which a flexible endoscope is inserted via the nose and the patient is asked to swallow different consistencies, visualizes directly the anatomy and function of the pharyngeal swallowing phase. Also, the sensory and motor components of swallowing can be assessed [44]. On the other hand, VFSS (also known as Modified Barium Swallow) provides information about the oral and oropharyngeal phases of the swallow, including dynamics of the swallowing process. With VFSS, it is possible to analyze the contact between the tongue base and posterior pharyngeal wall and it is more suitable for diagnosing aspiration during swallowing. VFSS is also more informative for detecting problems below the upper esophageal sphincter [45]. Preferably a VFSS is performed, to select eligible patients, but the choice of examination also depends upon clinical presentation, available instruments and clinician's preferences.

To visualize the potential injection sites in the oral cavity and pharynx the most crucial examination of the pre-lipofilling work-up is the Magnetic Resonance Imaging (MRI) [38]. Besides, with the MRI it is possible to evaluate the volume of the tongue and pharyngeal wall. In **Figure 2**, an MRI assessment pre- and post-lipofilling treatment is presented.

In addition to the objective assessments, it might also be helpful to explore patient-reported experiences. The MD Anderson Dysphagia Inventory (MDADI) [46] and the Swallowing Quality of Life questionnaire (SWAL-QOL) [47] are often used in HNC patients to analyze patients' reported swallowing-related quality of life.

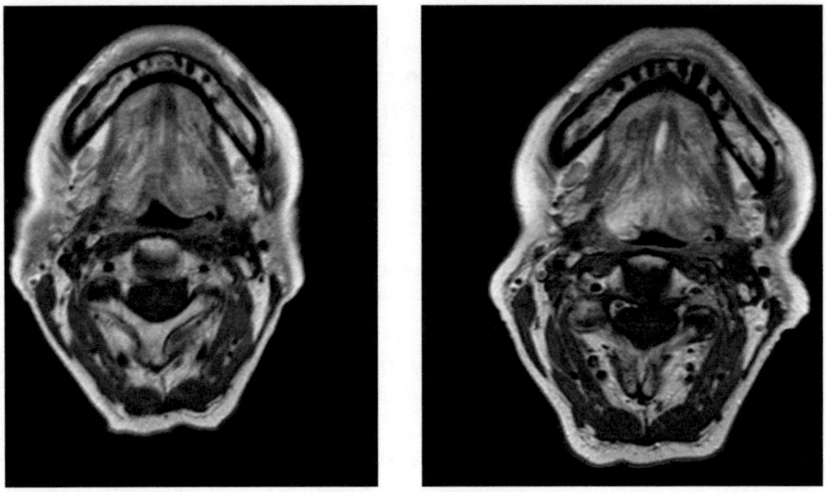

Figure 2.
MRI assessment pre- and post-lipofilling treatment. On the left side, the loss of tissue in the base of tongue is visible. On the right side, the base of tongue is larger and is filled up with fat.

4.3 Lipofilling procedure

Different techniques exist for lipofilling injection [41]. There are many preparation techniques for adipose tissue. There is no universally accepted standard method. The Coleman technique, which was described in the early 1990s, is the most frequently used method. This technique aims to prevent damage to the fragile adipose cells as much as possible during transplantation and thus promote tissue survival [48]. The technique involves three steps and is described by Hsu et al. [41]. The first step consists of the harvest of fatty tissue from the upper abdominal wall or inner thigh using large- or small-volume liposuction (see **Figure 3a**). The upper abdominal wall or lateral thigh is very useful as donor sites because of the high amount of local fat cells. The donor site can be infiltrated with tumescence fluid (for instance, ringers lactate, adrenaline and lidocaine) just before the liposuction, but this can also be done after the suction. After liposuction, the second step involves the preparation of the adipose tissue. During the preparation phase, the fat sample is transferred in a 10 cc syringe for centrifugation (see **Figure 3b**). The syringe is centrifuged for 2–3 minutes at 3000 rounds per minute (800 g) to separate out oils, debris, water (including lidocaine or adrenaline, saline and blood) and a layer of cell pellets/residue from the cellular fraction. In the syringe, three layers will be visible: the oil layer at the top, cellular fraction in the middle, and cellular debris and red blood cells at the bottom (see **Figure 3c**). The segregated cellular fraction, composed of adipocytes and stromal vascular cells, is transferred to a small 1 cc syringe. The third and last step consists of the injection into the predetermined spots in the base of the tongue. Using a needle, the side of the tongue is perforated, and the injection cannula is introduced. The dominant hand is used, or the injection is performed on cannula retraction in a three-dimensional "fan pattern." The aim is to transfer small aliquots of fat with multiple passes at different depths. The non-dominant fingers can be placed behind the tongue to control the process. It is helpful if the assistant pulls on the tongue (see **Figure 3d**). The same procedure is usually performed separately on both sides of the tongue. In general, we inject 10–15 cc of fat per session.

The lipofilling procedure can be carried out under local anesthesia or general anesthesia. Because 30–50% of the injected fat might be resorbed, and not too much fat can be injected at the same time, it is recommended to repeat the assessments,

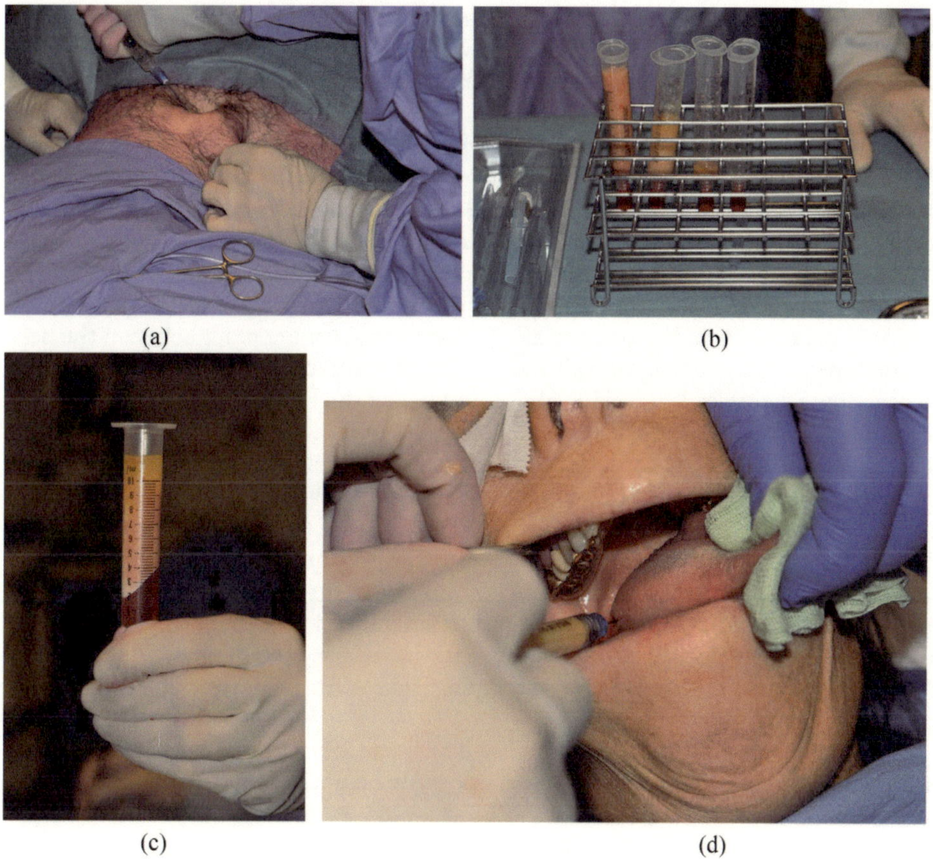

Figure 3.
The procedure of a lipofilling injection. (a) Fat harvest from the abdomen, (b) fat substance, (c) syringe with fat after centrifugation, (d) injecting fat into the base of tongue.

approximately 2–3 times. Preferably, between every injection procedure there is a period of 3 months to wait for the (positive) effect of the injection.

5. Short-term outcomes

In the last few years, different studies, primarily case reports, have been published about the use of lipofilling in patients with chronic dysphagia due to HNC (treatment) [38, 49, 50]. Navach et al. [49] reported about a 58-year-old patient with impaired swallowing after treatment for a nasopharyngeal carcinoma. This patient complained about dysphagia, the loss of body weight, aspiration pneumonia, and frequent episodes of bronchitis. A VFSS was conducted where a lack of bolus compression, asymmetry of the lingual movements, stagnation in the valleculae, lack of projection of the base of tongue, and more were visualized. The patient received 7 months of speech and language therapy to improve mobilization and strengthening of the swallowing muscles. The treatment improved the preparation and presentation of the bolus, although it was not sufficient enough. After 6 weeks, another VFSS showed a worsened bolus stagnation in the valleculae and at the base of tongue. This patient received a lipofilling injection in the base of tongue, which was performed following Coleman's procedure. In total, 5 cc of fat was injected into both sides of the base of tongue. After surgery, the patient experienced an improvement in swallowing, and minimal post-operative swelling was reported. A new VFSS was made 1 month after surgery, showing an improved swallowing mechanism due to greater elevation of the base of tongue, the effective elevation of the larynx, and an improved closure of the larynx. After 3 months, the swallowing function was still stable, and the patient gained body weight.

In our institute, a study was performed by Kraaijenga et al., to investigate the feasibility and potential value of lipofilling in HNC patients with post-treatment oropharyngeal dysfunction [38]. This case series included seven patients. One patient dropped out of the study because of progression and therefore, he chooses a total laryngectomy procedure. Pre-assessment of the six remaining patients included VFSS, MRI, and the SWAL-QOL measurements. VFSS showed penetration and/or aspiration in all but one patient. Reduced or absent contact between the base of the tongue and pharyngeal wall was seen in all six patients. This reduced or absent contact resulted in residue above and below the hyoid bone. MRI showed volume loss or atrophy of the tongue in five patients. Two patients had reduced tissue of the tonsillar in the right tonsillar arch. The lipofilling session was performed using the Coleman technique. Patients received two to three injection sessions at 3-month intervals. In total, 20–35 cc adipose tissue was transplanted in all patients. No complications, such as necrosis, infection, swelling, or edema, were observed. The follow-up took place 1–3 months post-surgery. VFSS showed that four patients had improved swallowing function, and two of them were no longer feeding tube dependent. The MRI showed increased tongue volume with the injected fat spread out at the base of tongue. The SWAL-QOL showed improved quality of life in almost all patients.

Recently, Ottaviani et al. [50] published a case report about a 76-year-old patient with severe chronic dysphagia who had undergone a horizontal supraglottic laryngectomy and adjuvant radiotherapy. FEES showed a mobile right arytenoid and tissue loss in the base of tongue. VFSS demonstrated constant intra-swallowing aspiration and moderate pooling of food at the base of tongue with post-swallowing penetration and aspiration. The patient received 6 months of speech therapy focused on muscle strengthening and postural compensation techniques. The intervention turned out insufficient, and therefore, lipofilling injection was offered as a treatment option. The surgery was performed following the Coleman technique, and 5 cc was injected into the base of tongue. Intraoperatively, FEES was performed and demonstrated an improved swallowing function. However, trace aspiration for liquid textures and minimal residue was seen. After 1 week, FEES demonstrated only aspiration for liquids. After 1 month, the VFSS showed mild to moderate dysphagia. These results were also stable at 6 months post-surgery.

These three studies showed that lipofilling might be an effective treatment for HNC patients with chronic dysphagia. No complications were reported, and therefore, lipofilling seems safe [38, 49, 50]. Many patients showed improved objective and subjective swallowing function after lipofilling. Nevertheless, it remains difficult to predict how much fat will be resorbed and thus how long a therapeutic effect will persist. With the Coleman technique, absorption of fat seems to be reduced to some extent [32, 33]. In general, after 20–30 cc injections (in 2–3 procedures), positive effects are seen. However, sometimes repeated injections might be needed to achieve and hold a therapeutic effect. Hopefully, the injected tissue may also become less fibrotic, and no further injections are needed. Until now, there is no large data available yet, supporting this hypothesis.

6. Case reports

To give a better insight into lipofilling and how it can be used in post-treatment swallowing problems in HNC patients, three cases will be described in detail (see

Case	Sex	Age	Tumor		Treatment	Lipofilling injections		
			Site	TNM		Site	No.	Amount (cc)
1	M	66	Oral cavity	T3N2c	Surgery + RT (1997)	Base of tongue	3	32.0
2	F	59	Base of tongue	T3N2c	CRT (2004)	Base of tongue	3	34.5
3	M	73	Hypo-pharynx	T2N1	CRT (1984)	Base of tongue	1	20.0

Abbreviations: M = male, F = female; TNM = classification of Malignant Tumors; RT = radiotherapy; CRT = chemo radiotherapy; No. = number of injections.

Table 1.
Characteristics of the three selected case reports.

Table 1). Patients' pre lipofilling objective and subjective swallowing function are analyzed and compared with the swallowing function after the last lipofilling (short-term results) and between 2.5 years and 5.8 years after the last lipofilling treatment (long-term results).

6.1 Case 1

A 67-year-old male, had been treated in 1997 for a T3N2c carcinoma of the floor of the mouth. His treatment consisted of local resection, partial mandibulectomy with free fibula reconstruction, and post-operative radiotherapy which resulted in complete remission. In 2013, 16 years after treatment, he visited the outpatient clinic with increasing swallowing difficulties, with particularly solid foods getting stuck in his throat, requiring placement of a PRG feeding tube to maintain adequate nutritional intake.

6.1.1 VFSS

VFSS assessments showed severe dysphagia with the occurrence of penetration and a high amount of oropharyngeal contrast residue due to insufficient contact between the base of tongue and posterior pharyngeal wall.

6.1.2 MRI

An MRI was made to rule out a new tumor. Since standard swallowing exercises for more than 1 year did not improve the persisting swallowing problems, and other surgical options were unlikely to improve the swallowing function. In **Figure 3**, the pre-lipofilling MRI scan can be found on the right.

6.1.3 Number of injections

This patient underwent three lipofilling sessions (3 times 8–12 cc) into the base of the tongue at 3-months intervals. After the second procedure, the patient noticed an improvement in swallowing function. He resumed oral intake following the third injection and his feeding tube could be removed.

6.1.4 Short-term results

A VFSS assessment showed improved scores for thick liquids (lower penetration and aspiration (PAS), see **Table 2**). This patient also reported notable improvement in subjective swallowing function, with substantially less effort and less choking. In **Figure 3**, the short-term post-lipofilling MRI scan is shown in the middle.

Case	Amount (cc)		FOIS	VFSS (PAS)			TL
				Thin	Thick	Solid	
1	32.0	Pre	3	4	4	3	No
		Post short*	6	4	2	3	
		Post long**	5	8	1	1	
2	34.5	Pre	1	NA	NA	NA	No
		Post short*	6	7	6	NA	
		Post long**	6	8	8	8	
3	20.0	Pre	1	7	5	NA	Yes
		Post	1	X	X	X	

Abbreviations: FOIS = functional oral intake scale: range 1–7, whereas 1 is 'no oral intake' and 7 means 'normal oral intake'; VFSS = video fluoroscopic swallowing study; PAS = penetration aspiration scale: range 1–8, lower scores mean better/safer swallowing function; TL = total laryngectomy; X = missing data; NA = not applicable (i.e., no transport possible); Post short = 1–3 months after lipofilling treatment; Post long** = up to 4 years after lipofilling treatment.*

Table 2.
Pre- and post-treatment outcomes after the lipofilling session.

6.1.5 Long-term results

However, 2.5 years later the SWAL-QOL subscale scores deteriorated (see **Table 3**). Until 2020, this patient was able to maintain oral intake without a PRG. Swallowing was not easy, but he managed to have a full oral intake with additional diet modifications. He died in 2020 due to urosepsis. In **Figure 4**, the long-term post-lipofilling MRI scan is shown on the right.

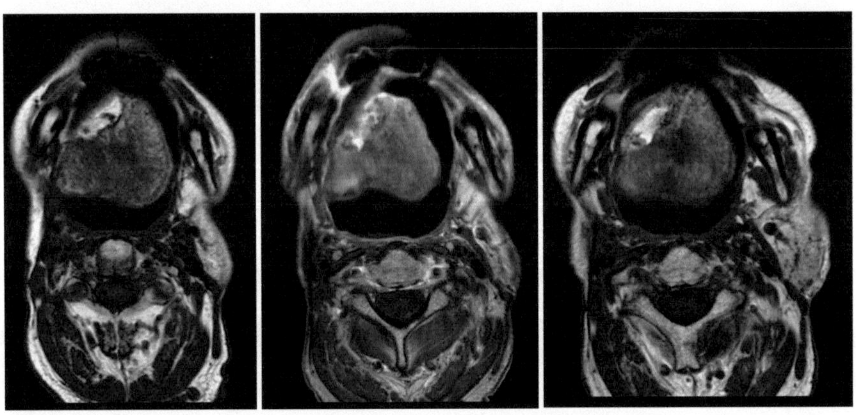

Figure 4.
MRI assessment of case 1 over time. On the left, pre-lipofilling injection. In the middle, short-term MRI (1-month post-treatment). On the right, long-term MRI (4 years post-treatment).

6.2 Case 2

A 59-year-old female, was diagnosed with a T3N2c base of tongue tumor in 2004. Organ-preservation treatment with concurrent chemo radiotherapy resulted in a complete remission. In the post-treatment period, however, the patient developed severe dysphagia and dysarthria due to oropharyngeal scarring and base of tongue atrophy. Despite intensive swallowing rehabilitation with strengthening exercises, several esophageal dilatations, and a customized intraoral prosthesis lowering the hard palate to also improve speech, the patient remained completely feeding tube dependent due to persistent oropharyngeal dysfunction/stagnation of food.

6.2.1 VFSS

VFSS evaluation demonstrated minimal contact between the base of tongue and the pharyngeal wall during swallowing, with large amounts of a residue located at the piriform sinus, and occurrence of aspiration, even at a 1 cc swallow administered with a pipet to improve bolus transport.

6.2.2 MRI

MRI showed an atrophic tongue, sagged posteriorly (see **Figure 5**). Since intensive swallowing exercises offered no solution, in 2014 the patient opted for lipofilling into the base of tongue.

6.2.3 Number of injections

Three lipofilling sessions were needed at 3-months intervals with 10–12 cc filled per session.

6.2.4 Short-term results

The post-operative MRI showed several fat depositions at the right base of the tongue (see **Figure 5**), and the patient was able to eat and drink again for the first time in 10 years. However, although the patient was very satisfied with being able to swallow again, the VFSS evaluation still showed aspiration. Four months later the patient presented with aspiration pneumonia, and a nasogastric feeding tube was indicated. However, although being aware of the possible risks, she chose to resume her per oral intake. At 8 months post-lipofilling (short-term results), she remained happy with the procedure resulting in good SWAL-QOL scores.

6.2.5 Long-term results

However, after 4 years of the last lipofilling this patient experienced more swallowing problems. Her subjective swallowing outcomes deteriorated (see Appendix, **Table 3** for her long-term SWAL-QOL scores) and she decided to have another lipofilling session. Nevertheless, even with that extra lipofilling (17 cc at the left and 17 cc at the right base of tongue) the SWAL-QOL scores increased meaning worse swallowing-related quality of life (see **Table 3** in the Appendix). In addition, the repeated VFSS showed worsening swallowing function (severe dysphagia). Since she was familiar with developing aspiration pneumonias, and weight loss, we decided to place a PRG and stop any oral intake. In **Figure 5**, the long-term MRI scan can be found on the right.

6.3 Case 3

A 73-year-old male, who had been diagnosed with a T2N1 hypopharynx carcinoma in 1984. He was treated with radiotherapy, which resulted in complete remission. This patient also had a history of esophageal carcinoma in 1964 for which he needed several dilatations in 1990/1991. Since 2009, he suffered from severe swallowing problems (several aspiration pneumonias) caused by a dysfunctional larynx and he needed a PRG.

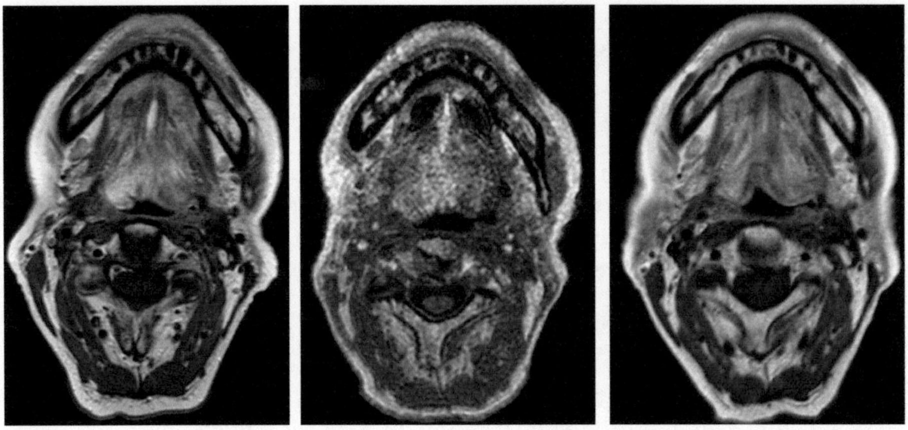

Figure 5.
MRI assessment of case 2 over time. On the left, pre-lipofilling injection. In the middle, short-term (after 3 months) MRI. On the right, long-term MRI (after 4 years).

6.3.1 VFSS

A VFSS showed a severe swallowing problem. All food consistencies were (silently) aspirated, the epiglottis was rigid, and the laryngeal elevation was limited. This patient started with intensive swallowing rehabilitation since he had had no swallowing exercises before. However, the rehabilitation did not improve the swallowing function enough to increase oral intake or to remove the PRG. In 2017, the patient opted for a lipofilling injection in the base of tongue.

6.3.2 Number of injections

In total 20 cc was injected, 10 cc on the left and 10 cc on the right.

6.3.3 Short-term results

After this first injection, the patient was still not able to swallow anything. He continued to develop pneumonias for which he used antibiotics daily. Because of the serious health risks related to the recurrent pneumonias, and his low swallowing related quality of life as measured by the SWAL-QOL (see **Table 3**), this patient decided to undergo a functional total laryngectomy in 2018.

7. Clinical implications

In our institute, the Netherlands Cancer Institute, lipofilling is considered as a safe procedure. Therefore, this procedure is embedded as standard care for specific swallowing therapy to refractory patients. When a patient visits the hospital with swallowing complaints, the first step is to start swallowing rehabilitation under the guidance of a specialized speech and language pathologist. If the swallowing exercises do not give a satisfactory result, lipofilling can be considered. Patients are eligible if they have severe dysphagia caused by volume loss or muscle atrophy of the tongue or pharyngeal musculature due to HNC treatment. Patients may be eligible if they have no history of major oral surgery.

In the past 5 years, 20 patients have been treated with lipofilling injections at our institute. The procedure is preferably performed in collaboration with the plastic surgeon and under complete anesthesia. We prefer general anesthesia because, in our experience, especially injecting the fat into the tongue felt uncomfortable. General anesthesia makes the injection less stressful for the patient. In general, we inject 10–15 cc of fat, and on average, two to three sessions are needed. No severe complications have been developed since we started performing this procedure.

8. Conclusions

This chapter describes the possible role of lipofilling in patients with chronic dysphagia after HNC treatment. Lipofilling is a technique for transplanting fat cells within one individual. This procedure has the potential to increase tissue volume and increase oropharyngeal function. Based on published results, the lipofilling technique seems to be safe and—in selected cases—of potential value for improving swallowing function in therapy-refractory HNC patients. For this reason, lipofilling should be considered as a treatment option for chronic dysphagia after HNC treatment.

Acknowledgements

We would like to thank S.A.C. (Sophie) Kraaijenga (MD, PhD) for her contribution regarding the collected pretreatment and early post treatment data, and A.F. (Anne) Kornman (SLP, MSc.) for her contribution with regard to updating all collected data.

Conflict of interest

The authors declare no conflict of interest.

Appendix

	SWAL-QOL								
	Case 1			Case 2			Case 3		
	Pre	Short	Long	Pre	Short	Long	Pre	Short	Long
General burden	88.0	25.0	100.0	13.0	0.0	25.0	50.0	75.0	X
Food selection	75.0	38.0	75.0	13.0	0.0	0.0	50.0	50.0	X
Eating duration	88.0	88.0	100.0	50.0	0.0	25.0	50.0	50.0	X
Eating desire	50.0	25.0	100.0	42.0	17.0	17.0	50.0	50.0	X
Fear of eating	56.0	63.0	56.0	38.0	0.0	44.0	56.0	63.0	X
Sleep	25.0	25.0	13.0	0.0	0.0	0.0	0.0	0.0	X
Fatigue	58.0	67.0	67.0	83.0	42.0	X	8.0	17.0	X
Communication	100.0	50.0	100.0	25.0	0.0	25.0	75.0	75.0	X
Mental health	45.0	35.0	30.0	40.0	0.0	X	50.0	50.0	X
Social function	55.0	55.0	75.0	30.0	20.0	X	35.0	60.0	X
Symptom scale	61.0	48.0	57.0	52.0	11.0	X	39.0	46.0	X

Abbreviations: SWAL-QOL = swallowing quality of life questionnaire: range 0–100; lower scores mean better subjective swallowing function. A difference score of 12 points or more was used to demonstrate improvement (+), deterioration (−), or equality (=). X = missing data.

Table 3.
SWAL-QOL scores pre and post (last) lipofilling of the three selected case reports.

Author details

Marise Neijman, R.T. Karsten, L. van der Molen, O. Lapid[2]
and M.W.M. van den Brekel[1,3]*

1 Netherlands Cancer Institute, Amsterdam, The Netherlands

2 Amsterdam University Medical Centre, University of Amsterdam, The Netherlands

3 University of Amsterdam, The Netherlands

*Address all correspondence to: m.vd.brekel@nki.nl

References

[1] Mody MD, Rocco JW, Yom SS, Haddad RI, Saba NF. Head and neck cancer. The Lancet. 2021;**398**(10318): 2289-99

[2] Blot WJ, McLaughlin JK, Winn DM, Austin DF, Greenberg RS, Preston-Martin S, et al. Smoking and drinking in relation to oral and pharyngeal cancer. Cancer Research. 1988;**48**(11):3282-3287

[3] Mehanna H, Beech T, Nicholson T, El-Hariry I, McConkey C, Paleri V, et al. Prevalence of human papillomavirus in oropharyngeal and nonoropharyngeal head and neck cancer—Systematic review and meta-analysis of trends by time and region. Head & Neck. 2013; **35**(5):747-755

[4] Chien YC, Chen JY, Liu MY, Yang HI, Hsu MM, Chen CJ, et al. Serologic markers of Epstein-Barr virus infection and nasopharyngeal carcinoma in Taiwanese men. The New England Journal of Medicine. 2001;**345**(26): 1877-1882

[5] Brierley JG, M. K.; Wittekind, Ch. TNM classification of malignant tumours. 8th ed. Oxford, UK; Hoboken, NJ: John Wiley & Sons, Inc.; 2017

[6] Hutcheson KA, Lewin JS, Barringer DA, Lisec A, Gunn GB, Moore MW, et al. Late dysphagia after radiotherapy-based treatment of head and neck cancer. Cancer. 2012;**118**(23): 5793-5799

[7] Lazarus C, Logemann JA, Pauloski BR, Rademaker AW, Helenowski IB, Vonesh EF, et al. Effects of radiotherapy with or without chemotherapy on tongue strength and swallowing in patients with oral cancer. Head & Neck. 2007;**29**(7):632-637

[8] Mortensen HR, Jensen K, Aksglaede K, Behrens M, Grau C. Late dysphagia after IMRT for head and neck cancer and correlation with dose-volume parameters. Radiotherapy and Oncology. 2013;**107**(3):288-294

[9] Metreau A, Louvel G, Godey B, Le Clech G, Jegoux F. Long-term functional and quality of life evaluation after treatment for advanced pharyngolaryngeal carcinoma. Head & Neck. 2014;**36**(11):1604-1610

[10] Hutcheson KA, Bhayani MK, Beadle BM, Gold KA, Shinn EH, Lai SY, et al. Eat and exercise during radiotherapy or chemoradiotherapy for pharyngeal cancers: Use it or lose it. JAMA Otolaryngology. Head & Neck Surgery. 2013;**139**(11):1127-1134

[11] Garcia-Peris P, Paron L, Velasco C, de la Cuerda C, Camblor M, Breton I, et al. Long-term prevalence of oropharyngeal dysphagia in head and neck cancer patients: Impact on quality of life. Clinical Nutrition. 2007;**26**(6):710-717

[12] Langendijk JA, Doornaert P, Verdonck-de Leeuw IM, Leemans CR, Aaronson NK, Slotman BJ. Impact of late treatment-related toxicity on quality of life among patients with head and neck cancer treated with radiotherapy. Journal of Clinical Oncology. 2008;**26**(22):3770-3776

[13] Passchier E, Stuiver MM, van der Molen L, Kerkhof SI, van den Brekel MW, Hilgers FJ. Feasibility and impact of a dedicated multidisciplinary rehabilitation program on health-related quality of life in advanced head and neck cancer patients. European Archives of Oto-Rhino-Laryngology. 2016;**273**(6):1577-1587

[14] Eades M, Murphy J, Carney S, Amdouni S, Lemoignan J, Jelowicki M, et al. Effect of an interdisciplinary rehabilitation program on quality of life in patients with head and neck cancer:

Review of clinical experience. Head & Neck. 2013;**35**(3):343-349

[15] van der Molen L, van Rossum MA, Burkhead LM, Smeele LE, Rasch CR, Hilgers FJ. A randomized preventive rehabilitation trial in advanced head and neck cancer patients treated with chemoradiotherapy: Feasibility, compliance, and short-term effects. Dysphagia. 2011;**26**(2):155-170

[16] Retel VP, van der Molen L, Hilgers FJ, Rasch CR, L'Ortye AA, Steuten LM, et al. A cost-effectiveness analysis of a preventive exercise program for patients with advanced head and neck cancer treated with concomitant chemo-radiotherapy. BMC Cancer. 2011;**11**:475

[17] Kotz T, Federman AD, Kao J, Milman L, Packer S, Lopez-Prieto C, et al. Prophylactic swallowing exercises in patients with head and neck cancer undergoing chemoradiation: A randomized trial. Archives of Otolaryngology—Head & Neck Surgery. 2012;**138**(4):376-382

[18] Carnaby-Mann G, Crary MA, Schmalfuss I, Amdur R. "Pharyngocise": Randomized controlled trial of preventative exercises to maintain muscle structure and swallowing function during head-and-neck chemoradiotherapy. International Journal of Radiation Oncology, Biology, Physics. 2012;**83**(1):210-219

[19] Carroll WR, Locher JL, Canon CL, Bohannon IA, McColloch NL, Magnuson JS. Pretreatment swallowing exercises improve swallow function after chemoradiation. The Laryngoscope. 2008;**118**(1):39-43

[20] Kulbersh BD, Rosenthal EL, McGrew BM, Duncan RD, McColloch NL, Carroll WR, et al. Pretreatment, preoperative swallowing exercises may improve dysphagia quality of life. The Laryngoscope. 2006;**116**(6):883-886

[21] van der Molen L, van Rossum MA, Rasch CR, Smeele LE, Hilgers FJ. Two-year results of a prospective preventive swallowing rehabilitation trial in patients treated with chemoradiation for advanced head and neck cancer. European Archives of Oto-Rhino-Laryngology. 2014;**271**(5):1257-1270

[22] Bhayani MK, Hutcheson KA, Barringer DA, Lisec A, Alvarez CP, Roberts DB, et al. Gastrostomy tube placement in patients with oropharyngeal carcinoma treated with radiotherapy or chemoradiotherapy: Factors affecting placement and dependence. Head & Neck. 2013;**35**(11):1634-1640

[23] Logemann JA, Pauloski BR, Rademaker AW, Colangelo LA. Super-supraglottic swallow in irradiated head and neck cancer patients. Head & Neck. 1997;**19**(6):535-540

[24] Lazarus C, Logemann JA, Gibbons P. Effects of maneuvers on swallowing function in a dysphagic oral cancer patient. Head & Neck. 1993;**15**(5):419-424

[25] Hind JA, Nicosia MA, Roecker EB, Carnes ML, Robbins J. Comparison of effortful and noneffortful swallows in healthy middle-aged and older adults. Archives of Physical Medicine and Rehabilitation. 2001;**82**(12):1661-1665

[26] Kahrilas PJ, Logemann JA, Krugler C, Flanagan E. Volitional augmentation of upper esophageal sphincter opening during swallowing. The American Journal of Physiology. 1991;**260**(3 Pt 1):G450-G456

[27] Lazarus C, Logemann JA, Song CW, Rademaker AW, Kahrilas PJ. Effects of voluntary maneuvers on tongue base function for swallowing. Folia

Phoniatrica et Logopaedica. 2002;**54**(4): 171-176

[28] Shaker R, Kern M, Bardan E, Taylor A, Stewart ET, Hoffmann RG, et al. Augmentation of deglutitive upper esophageal sphincter opening in the elderly by exercise. The American Journal of Physiology. 1997;**272**(6 Pt 1): G1518-G1522

[29] Kraaijenga SA, van der Molen L, Stuiver MM, Teertstra HJ, Hilgers FJ, van den Brekel MW. Effects of strengthening exercises on swallowing musculature and function in senior healthy subjects: A prospective effectiveness and feasibility study. Dysphagia. 2015;**30**(4):392-403

[30] Kraaijenga SAC, Molen LV, Stuiver MM, Takes RP, Al-Mamgani A, Brekel M, et al. Efficacy of a novel swallowing exercise program for chronic dysphagia in long-term head and neck cancer survivors. Head & Neck. 2017;**39**(10):1943-1961

[31] Karsten RT, Ter Beek LC, Jasperse B, van Alphen MJA, Peeters JM, van der Molen L, et al. MRI assessment of swallow muscle activation with the swallow exercise aid and with conventional exercises in healthy volunteers: An explorative biomechanical study. Dysphagia. 2021; **36**(1):41-53

[32] Hoesseini A, Honings J, Taus-Mohamedradja R, van den Hoogen FJ, Marres HA, van den Broek GB, et al. Outcomes of endoscopic cricopharyngeal myotomy with CO_2 laser surgery: A retrospective study of 47 patients. Head & Neck. 2016;**38**(7): 1022-1027

[33] Qu SH, Li M, Liang JP, Su ZZ, Chen SQ, He XG. Laryngotracheal closure and cricopharyngeal myotomy for intractable aspiration and dysphagia secondary to cerebrovascular accident. ORL: Journal for Otorhinolaryngology and Its Related Specialties. 2009;**71**(6): 299-304

[34] Ahsan SF, Meleca RJ, Dworkin JP. Botulinum toxin injection of the cricopharyngeus muscle for the treatment of dysphagia. Otolaryngology and Head and Neck Surgery. 2000; **122**(5):691-695

[35] Zaninotto G, Marchese Ragona R, Briani C, Costantini M, Rizzetto C, Portale G, et al. The role of botulinum toxin injection and upper esophageal sphincter myotomy in treating oropharyngeal dysphagia. Journal of Gastrointestinal Surgery. 2004;**8**(8): 997-1006

[36] Theunissen EA, Timmermans AJ, Zuur CL, Hamming-Vrieze O, Paul de Boer J, Hilgers FJ, et al. Total laryngectomy for a dysfunctional larynx after (chemo)radiotherapy. Archives of Otolaryngology—Head & Neck Surgery. 2012;**138**(6):548-555

[37] Kos MP, David EF, Aalders IJ, Smit CF, Mahieu HF. Long-term results of laryngeal suspension and upper esophageal sphincter myotomy as treatment for life-threatening aspiration. The Annals of Otology, Rhinology, and Laryngology. 2008; **117**(8):574-580

[38] Kraaijenga SA, Lapid O, van der Molen L, Hilgers FJ, Smeele LE, van den Brekel MW. Feasibility and potential value of lipofilling in post-treatment oropharyngeal dysfunction. The Laryngoscope. 2016;**126**(12):2672-2678

[39] Van de Graaf R, Korteweg S. Gustav Adolf Neuber (1850-1932) and the first report on fat auto-grafting in humans in 1893. History Plastic Surgery. 2010;**1**(1): 7-11

[40] Hammond SE, Samuels S, Thaller S. Filling in the Details: A Review of Lipofilling of Radiated Tissues in the Head and Neck. The Journal of

Craniofacial Surgery. 2019;**30**(3): 667-671

[41] Hsu VM, Stransky CA, Bucky LP, Percec I. Fat grafting's past, present, and future: Why adipose tissue is emerging as a critical link to the advancement of regenerative medicine. Aesthetic Surgery Journal. 2012;**32**(7):892-899

[42] Krastev TK, Schop SJ, Hommes J, Piatkowski A, van der Hulst R. Autologous fat transfer to treat fibrosis and scar-related conditions: A systematic review and meta-analysis. Journal of Plastic, Reconstructive & Aesthetic Surgery. 2020;**73**(11):2033-2048

[43] Negenborn VL, Groen JW, Smit JM, Niessen FB, Mullender MG. The use of autologous fat grafting for treatment of scar tissue and scar-related conditions: A systematic review. Plastic and Reconstructive Surgery. 2016;**137**(1): 31e-43e

[44] Leder SB, Murray JT. Fiberoptic endoscopic evaluation of swallowing. Physical Medicine and Rehabilitation Clinics of North America. 2008;**19**(4): 787-801, viii-ix

[45] Giraldo-Cadavid LF, Leal-Leano LR, Leon-Basantes GA, Bastidas AR, Garcia R, Ovalle S, et al. Accuracy of endoscopic and videofluoroscopic evaluations of swallowing for oropharyngeal dysphagia. The Laryngoscope. 2017;**127**(9):2002-2010

[46] Chen AY, Frankowski R, Bishop-Leone J, Hebert T, Leyk S, Lewin J, et al. The development and validation of a dysphagia-specific quality-of-life questionnaire for patients with head and neck cancer: The M.D. Anderson dysphagia inventory. Archives of Otolaryngology—Head & Neck Surgery. 2001;**127**(7):870-876

[47] McHorney CA, Robbins J, Lomax K, Rosenbek JC, Chignell K, Kramer AE, et al. The SWAL-QOL and SWAL-CARE outcomes tool for oropharyngeal dysphagia in adults: III. Documentation of reliability and validity. Dysphagia. 2002;**17**(2):97-114

[48] Pu LLQ, Coleman SR, Cui X, Ferguson REH Jr, Vasconez HC. Autologous fat grafts harvested and refined by the Coleman technique: A comparative study. Plastic and Reconstructive Surgery. 2008;**122**(3): 932-937

[49] Navach V, Calabrese LS, Zurlo V, Alterio D, Funicelli L, Giugliano G. Functional base of tongue fat injection in a patient with severe postradiation dysphagia. Dysphagia. 2011;**26**(2): 196-199

[50] Ottaviani F, Schindler A, Klinger F, Scarponi L, Succo G, Mozzanica F. Functional fat injection under local anesthesia to treat severe postsurgical dysphagia, case report. Head & Neck. 2019;**41**(1):E17-E21

Chapter 8

Introducing IQoro: A Clinically Effective Oral Neuromuscular Treatment for Dysphagia

Mary Hägg and Natalie R. Morris

Abstract

There is a clear need for new advances in treating dysphagia; healthcare professionals currently have a restricted range of options to treat swallowing problems and related conditions. Usual treatments for dysphagia are based on compensatory measures which allow patients to live within the limitations of their condition. These measures do not address the underlying cause of dysphagia: neurological and physiological dysfunction. A senior speech and language therapist working with young people with Cerebral Palsy bemoans the fact that official care pathway guidelines list only medication and surgical intervention as alternatives to treat drooling. Neither of which, she contends, is effective or desirable. Esophageal dysphagia causes reflux-based diseases, which are also poorly served by current treatment alternatives and are currently managed by medication, or remedied by surgical intervention. Medication reduces the symptoms of reflux but does nothing to address the underlying pathophysiology, muscular dysfunction, at the root of the problem. That now changes with IQoro: a simple, innovative treatment that is available to patients and healthcare professionals to address all of the above conditions. The chapter explains the physiological and neurological process of the functional swallow in detail, with illustrations and explanations. The efficacy of IQoro treatment is proven with evidence from internationally published scientific studies, case studies, an NHS service evaluation, and NICE briefings.

Keywords: oropharyngeal dysphagia, esophageal dysphagia, reflux, hiatal hernia, neuromuscular training, cerebral palsy, service evaluation in NHS, NICE briefing

1. Introduction

Dysphagia is a widely prevalent phenomenon that brings the risk of other conditions like malnutrition, pneumonia, and even the necessity for non-oral feeding solutions [1–3]. It always leads to reduced quality of life, and can even be fatal [4].

1.1 Few real solutions

The ways that patients with dysphagia are cared for fall into two broad categories, of which the first is by far the most common. Patients are often provided with compensatory care, [5, 6] which allows them to live with the disabilities that dysphagia brings. These therapies may include modified often puréed solid foods that are easier to swallow, and thickened drinks that can be swallowed more safely with less risk of aspiration. Instruction on posture, eating habits, oral hygiene and more, are also common.

The second category of care is rehabilitation treatment [7–11] to address the causes of the dysphagia. In general they focus on increasing muscle strength in the affected organs.

1.2 A new, innovative solution

This chapter introduces a simple neuromuscular treatment using an oral therapy - IQoro (**Figure 1**) - that can usually be self-administered by the patient. The treatment has clinical evidence and scientific proof of striking success in treating people of all ages with all forms of dysphagia: oral-, pharyngeal- and esophageal [12–14]. When used with stroke survivors, the research shows equally good outcomes regardless of whether treatment started immediately, or long after the onset of stroke [10]. In scientific studies, the observed improved outcomes were still present at long-term follow-ups performed up to 18 months after the end of treatment [11, 12, 15–17].

2. Two innovative clinicians

2.1 Mary's journey

Associate professor Mary Hägg started her professional life as a hospital dentist where she became fascinated with the swallowing problems that some of her patients presented with. In Sweden, the remit of the dentist is wider than in some other countries and can encompass more orofacial issues than just teeth and gums. The more she worked with patients with swallowing difficulties some after stroke the more fascinated she became. She worked with exercises to strengthen the delinquent muscles and became more and more renowned for her focus on dysphagia.

In 1990, Mary founded a specialist multi-disciplinary unit within the ENT department of a Swedish teaching hospital and has managed it since its inception. The purpose of this speech and the swallowing unit is to encourage and ensure cooperation across a range of clinical specialties to deliver improved patient outcomes.

In 1997 she was awarded a stipend to visit and study the subject more deeply with Dr. Castillo Morales, Cordoba, Argentina, and in 2001 with Professor Bronwyn Jones, Dept. of Radiology, The Johns Hopkins Hospital, medical center in Baltimore, Maryland, USA.

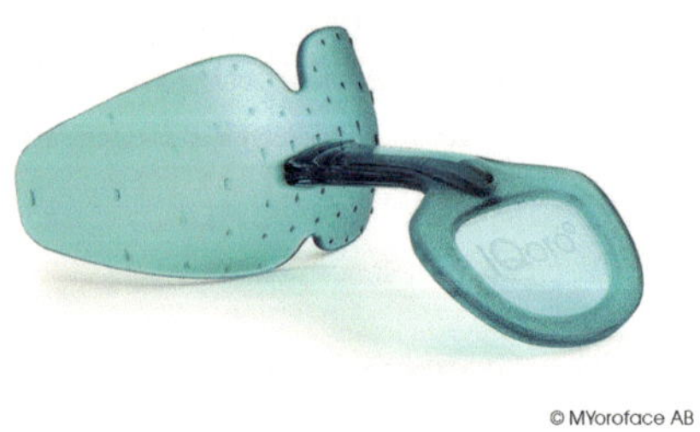

Figure 1.
The IQoro neuromuscular training device.

As she treated more and more patients that were referred to her, she came to two conclusions: firstly, those swallowing difficulties manifest themselves as a muscular deficiency, but usually have a neurological dysfunction at the root; and secondly, that there were few effective treatment options. In many cases, patients received only compensatory care which allowed them to function with their disability, but with no active plan to address the underlying problem.

To address the first issue Mary decided that she must study to be a doctor in order to understand the neurology that lies behind dysphagia. It is clear that the day before a patient has a stroke that his or her swallowing can be fine and that it is the neurological event that causes the immediate onset of dysphagia. Mary's Ph.D. thesis "Sensory-motor brain plasticity in stroke patients with dysphagia. A methodological study on investigation and treatment" 2007, used massage to restore muscular strength by stimulating brain activity. Mary invented and had manufactured a validated scientific instrument to measure the strength of certain components in the swallowing chain by measuring resistance in the pharyngeal sling or buccinator mechanism [18, 19]. She also developed and validated orofacial motor test methodologies [20].

The second problem, the lack of suitable treatments [21, 22] that could be easily and widely used even by the patients themselves was a harder task. Her journey took her through working with all types of dysphagia in people from premature babies through children, adults, and to end-of-life. The journey resulted in her inventing, developing, and patenting the revolutionary IQoro device that is now, July 2021, used by over 50,000 people in many countries.

2.2 Natalie's vision

Decades later Natalie Morris came across the IQoro device, and it set her wondering if it would help her patients too. Natalie is a Speech and Language Therapist working in the UK and is the founder and CEO of The Feeding Trust a not-for-profit multi-disciplinary feeding clinic in the Midlands. During her 20-year career as an SLT, Natalie has become specialist in the assessment and treatment of communication and swallowing difficulties in children and young people (CYP) with neuro-developmental disabilities and acquired brain injuries. She is the founder of Integrated Therapy Solutions Ltd. where she and her team help CYP with swallowing difficulties.

She looked at the scientific evidence supporting IQoro and was disappointed to find that there was none that was directly relevant to one of her main patient groups: CYP clients with Cerebral Palsy (CP). This was significant because NICE guidelines for the management of saliva control in CP [23] offer few options:

1. Assess contributory factors before starting drug therapy

2. Medication

3. Botulinum toxin injections

4. Surgery

In other words, the only treatment options after considering compensatory strategies such as positioning, are drug therapy or surgery. But the Cochrane review of interventions for drooling in children with CP according to Walshe M, Smith M, Pennington L 2012 [24] concludes: "*There is no clear consensus on which interventions are safe and effective in managing drooling in children with CP.*" Her own clinical observations and experiences over the years have been that difficulties with saliva control are a persistent problem with no real effective treatment.

Natalie reasoned that if IQoro could help patients with neurological problems such as after a stroke, then it might help her patients with CP too. And if there was no evidence to prove that it worked, then she would have to investigate it herself.

This chapter will show the success of these two clinicians' work.

3. The physiology of the swallow

This is a brief description of the four different physiological phases of the swallowing process, the following section will look at the neurology of the swallow in detail [5, 25].

During a day, a normal person swallows approximately 600 times: 350 of these are during the day, 200 when eating or drinking, and 50 times when asleep. We use our voluntary muscles to transfer food to our mouths and chew it, after this our reflexive systems take over to complete the swallow unconsciously. When we swallow whilst asleep it is, of course, an entirely reflexive process.

3.1 The phases of the swallow

3.1.1 Pre-oral phase

Simply described, the swallowing process starts when we transfer food from the plate to the mouth (**Figure 2**). This phase is negatively affected when postural control or arm and hand motility are reduced, possibly after stroke [17].

3.1.2 Oral phase

The oral phase (**Figure 2**) starts when we close our lips, chew, reduce the food to manageable pieces and mix it with saliva. As the food is formed into a bolus the tongue's backward and upwards movements propel it towards the pharynx, at the same time the floor of the mouth rises. And then immediately before the swallowing reflex is triggered we press our lips together creating a low pressure in the mouth. This activity normally takes up to 10 seconds [5]. The decrease in pressure in the mouth eases the transport of the food mixture from the mouth to the pharynx.

The phases employ a mixture of voluntary and involuntary commands.

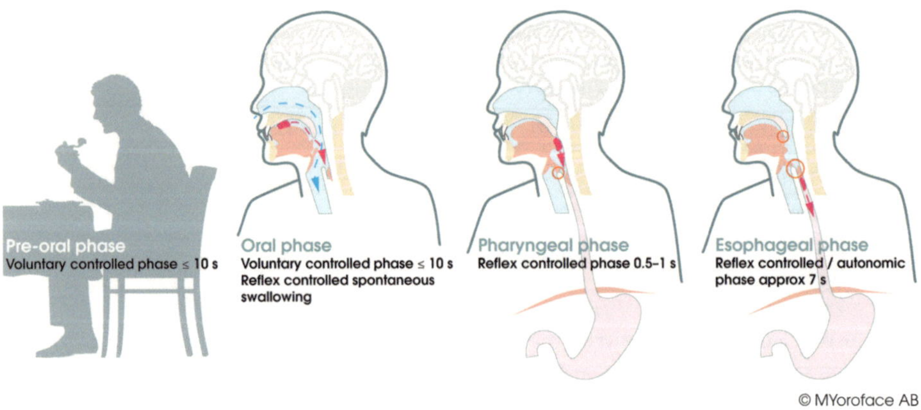

Figure 2.
The four phases of the swallowing process.

3.1.3 Pharyngeal phase

Once the bolus has passed the anterior palatal arch towards the pharynx, the swallow reflex takes over. This is controlled by the brain stem no longer consciously controlled as the pre-oral and oral phases were. The interplay between the voluntary and involuntary processes is described in the following section on the neurology of the swallow.

A normal swallow requires a balance between the infrahyoid and suprahyoid muscles to stimulate the swallowing reflex [20, 26].

In a later section "The neurology of the swallow" we will see that these muscles are triggered by the following nerves - Infrahyoidal muscles: CN XII hypoglossus.

– Suprahyoidal muscles: CN VII facialis, CN V trigeminus, CN XII hypoglossus.

Middle illustration: A Functional swallow is prepared when the hyoid bone is pulled backward and upwards (red arrow) by the styloid muscles (CN VII) and the posterior part of the digastric muscles (CN VII), at the same moment as the tongue base retracts.

The swallow reflex is then triggered when the hyoid bone is pulled forwards and upwards (blue arrow) by the digastricus anterior abdomen (CN V), m. mylohyoideus (CN V), and m. geniohyoideus (CN XII). At the same moment, a breathing suspension is caused as the epiglottis closes the laryngeal air pathway, and tongue forward movement is initiated. The chewing muscles are active throughout the swallow.

Left illustration: A dysfunctional swallow. If the chewing muscles are weak, the patient cannot lift his lower jaw and close his lips fully, which hinders swallowing. At the same time, the lower muscle groups of the tongue pull the hyoid bone downwards, which further degrades swallowing ability. The same thing happens when grinding the teeth.

Right illustration: A dysfunctional swallow. When the head falls backward, because of impaired head control, the mouth opens spontaneously and the equilibrium of the hyoid bone is completely upset, resulting in swallowing difficulties.

The pharyngeal phase (**Figures 2–4**) is a critical part of the swallow controlled purely reflexively and takes between 0.5 and 1 second. It requires a precise interplay between breathing and swallowing functions [5, 13]. When the bolus is to be swallowed, the tongue moves it back towards the anterior palatal arch and the

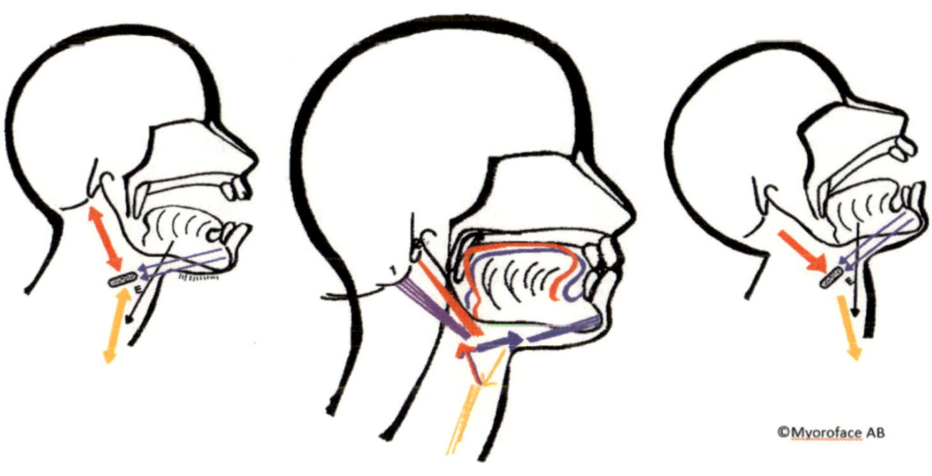

Figure 3.
Functional and dysfunctional swallow.

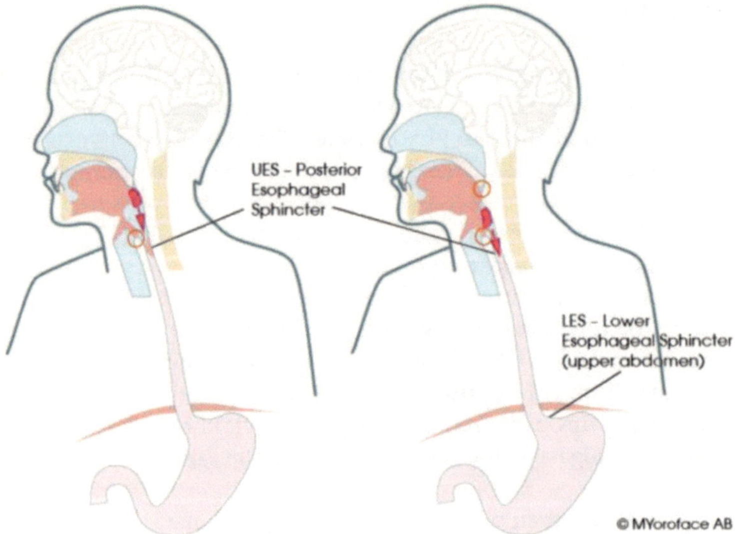

Figure 4.
The pharyngeal phase - a critical phase requiring coordination of swallowing and breathing.

smooth palate which seals against the nasal passages. The larynx raises reflexively, and the tongue starts its forward movement.

The first of four security levels to prevent aspiration of food or drink is now activated. The constrictor muscles: *Constrictor pharyngeus superior*, *Constrictor pharyngeus middle*, *Constrictor pharyngeus inferior* contract [27]. The last of these is also known as the UES [28]. The second level is achieved when the epiglottis closes over the trachea or air pathway. The third and fourth levels are executed as first the false vocal cords close, and then the true vocal cords themselves.

There is perhaps more crossover in dysfunction in the different phases than is often thought. Misdiagnosis is a risk when healthcare professionals concentrate too much on their own specialities without considering a more holistic approach.

For example:

- Mis-directed swallowing, post-nasal drip, aspiration, hoarse or gurgly voice, persistent non-productive cough, something stuck in the throat, and blockage are all symptoms often thought of as being caused by a brain injury. Causes of such brain damage can be a stroke, trauma, progressive neurological diseases, or other. In fact, all the symptoms described could equally well be caused by a Hiatal hernia [14].

- Patients exhibiting voice changes are often referred in firsthand to a speech and language therapist. If the SLT is not aware that the cause of the problem may be dysfunction in the esophageal phase - like a Hiatal hernia - then optimal outcomes may not be achieved. This problem is aggravated by the fact that SLTs in some countries are not routinely concerned with esophageal dysfunction.

- Patients with symptoms of Hiatal hernia are often referred to a medical consultant to rule out the possibility of stroke. When this has been done, then the finger may be pointed at a brain tumor, ALS, or some other neurological condition. Examination for these conditions is both alarming for the patient whilst waiting for examination and results, and expensive. Around 20% of the world's population suffers from a reflux-based condition, and it is thus logical in many cases to start treating for a Hiatal hernia as soon as stroke has been ruled out.

3.1.4 Esophageal phase

The esophageal phase (**Figure 2**) concerns the movement of food and drink from the esophagus down to the stomach. The esophagus' longitudinal musculature is activated, forming a stiff pipe and allowing the entrance to the Upper Esophageal Sphincter (UES) to relax and open to allow the passage of the bolus into the esophagus. At the same time, the Lower Esophageal Sphincter (LES) opens to allow the entrance of the bolus to the stomach [5, 29]. This phase takes around 7 seconds to complete.

As well as the outer longitudinal layer of muscles, the esophagus also has an inner layer of circular muscles. To transport the food down to the stomach, these circular muscles produce coordinated peristaltic wave motions - this explains why we can swallow even if we were hanging upside down.

4. The neurology of the swallow

4.1 The phases of the swallow

The four phases of the swallowing process described above involve 148 muscles and six cranial nerves. Of course, the muscular activities described are not separate from the nerve and brain activity that control them, the entire neurophysiology [25] of the swallowing process must work correctly. Understanding how is fundamental to appreciating how a dysfunctional swallow can be treated.

Figure 5 illustrates four important areas of the brain [25].

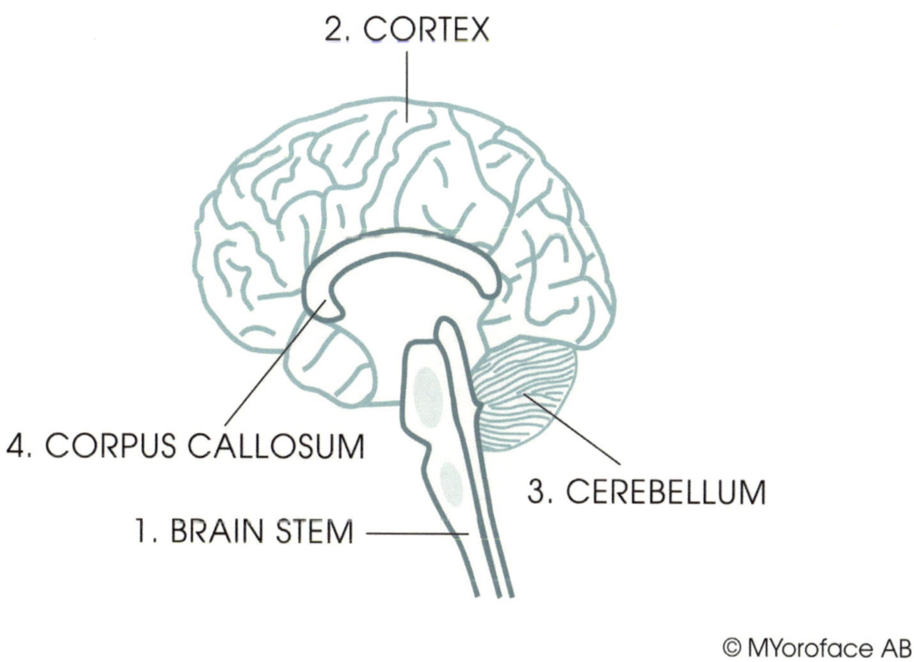

Figure 5.
The brain.

1. Brain stem: It controls non-voluntary "unconscious" automatic functions such as breathing, blood pressure, heart rhythm, the reflex swallowing phases; and also functions as a communication node between the cerebrum, the cerebellum, the spinal cord, and the peripheral nervous system.

2. Cortex: It controls our voluntary "conscious" most advanced functions such as language, thinking, fine-motor skills, and the voluntary swallowing phases.

3. Cerebellum: It co-ordinates our movements, our balance, and our ability to act in response to our immediate surroundings.

4. Corpus callosum: It connects the two brain hemispheres' cortex areas with each other. It consists of some 200 to 800 million nerves that coordinate the activities of the brain's two hemispheres.

4.2 Brain functions in swallowing

The sensory nerves report perceptions of pressure, texture, taste, and temperature, and these are transmitted by these afferent nerves to the brain. The primary source of these stimuli is from the nerves in the lips and then, in turn, the tongue, soft palate, and pharynx (**Figure 6**) [5, 29]. The (CN V) Trigeminus is the thickest and fastest of the efferent nerves, and thus the signals from the lips are the first to reach the brain stem. It is therefore a mistake to concentrate on therapies for the tongue, soft palate, and pharynx that omit the importance of the lips.

The five cranial motor nerves that are important for swallowing are CN V Trigeminus, CN VII Facialis, CN IX Glossopharyngeus, CN X, Vagus, and CN XII Hypoglossus. The first four are both sensory (afferent), and motor (efferent) nerve pathways; which send information both to and from the brain - the sensory-motoric reflex arc.

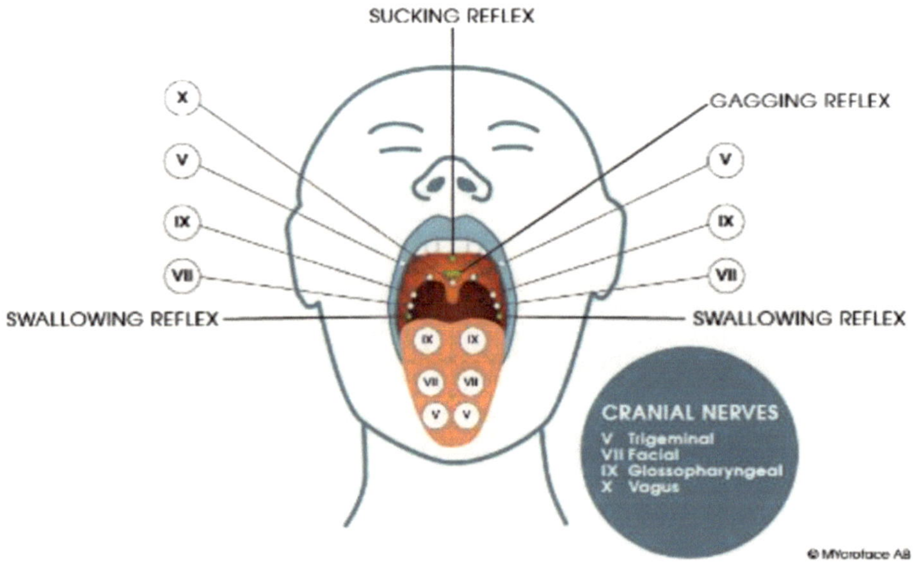

Figure 6.
The cranial nerves and reflex points of the oral cavity.

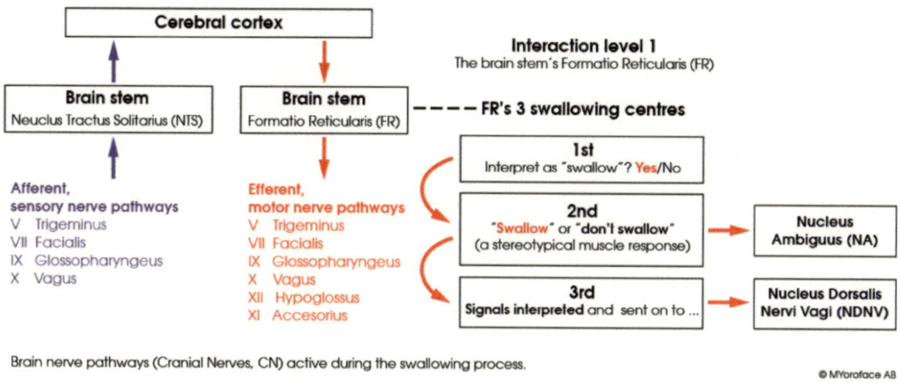

Figure 7.
The sensory-motor reflex arc (level 1).

In the brain stem (**Figure 7**) we find the Nucleus Tractus Solitarius (NTS): the afferent nucleus. The NTS is the core that gathers all incoming sensory signals via the afferent nerve pathways as described (**Figure 7**). The NTS then transmits the signals onwards either to the brain's cortex or directly to the network-like system in the brainstem called the Formatio Reticularis (FR). These efferent motor signals are transmitted to the musculature of the face, mouth, esophagus, diaphragm, down to the stomach, the intestines, and the rectum. The process by which the incoming sensory signals trigger afferent commands is known as the sensory-motoric reflex arc (**Figure 7**) [5, 25, 26, 29].

The three swallowing centers' interactions - from the brain stem to muscles.

In the FR, the afferent signals from the NTS and the cortex (**Figure 7**) are first interpreted and then passed through various distribution nodes to the efferent nuclei: the Nucleus Ambiguus (NA), and the Nucleus Dorsalis Nervi Vagi (NDNV).

The NA (**Figure 7**) sends impulses to the skeletally striated musculature in the oral and pharyngeal regions; and the NDNV (**Figure 7**) to the smooth musculature of the esophagus and beyond. How these function during swallowing we will explain in more detail below.

In the FR there are three distribution nodes (swallowing centers) that are key to the swallowing process; as well as a number of other centers that control breathing, speech, chewing, coughing, vomiting, evacuation of the bowels and bladder, and those muscles that control the body's posture (**Figure 8**). [5, 25, 26, 29].

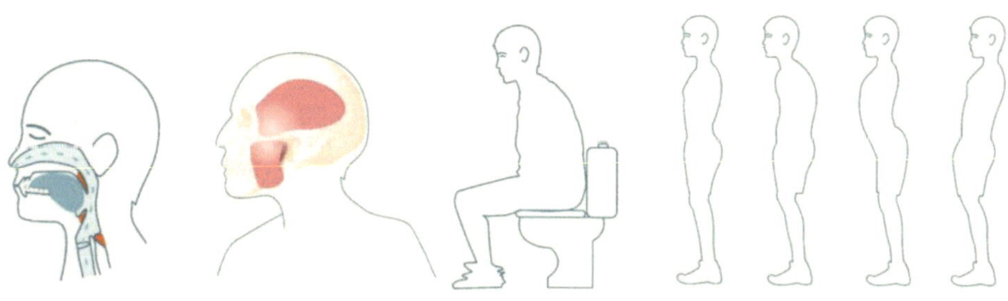

Figure 8.
The Formatio Reticularis (FR) is the control centre for a variety of vital functions.

The Formatio Reticularis is the control centre for several vital functions including breathing, speech, chewing, coughing, vomiting, evacuation of the bowels and bladder, and those muscles that control the body's posture.

The incoming information is routed by the Nucleus Tractus Solitarius (NTS) in two pathways: some directly to the first of the three swallowing centers in the brain stem, whilst the remainder of the information continues upwards to the cortex to be processed before being also directed to the first swallowing center (**Figure** 7).

4.3 The swallowing centers

4.3.1 First swallowing center

If the combination of information received by the first swallowing center (**Figure 9**) from the NTS and from the cortex is interpreted as that something is to be swallowed, this instruction is sent to the second swallowing center.

4.3.2 Second swallowing center

The second swallowing center (**Figure 9**) transmits signals to the muscles via the motor nerves – the downward-transmitting efferent nerve pathways. Here, there is a pre-programmed "swallow / don't swallow" stereotypical muscle response.

If the food is to be swallowed, a command is sent to the NA, which in its turn sends the instruction via the efferent nerve pathways to the striated musculature in the oral and pharyngeal regions of the swallowing chain. Concurrently, impulses are also sent to the third swallowing center.

4.3.3 Third swallowing center

The third swallowing center (**Figure 9**) transmits information to the NDNV - an efferent nucleus and then onwards to the esophagus' smooth musculature to complete the swallowing action and to transport the bolus downwards to the stomach.

The three swallowing centers' interactions from the 2nd center to the striated muscles, and the 3rd center to the smooth muscles is illustrated here.

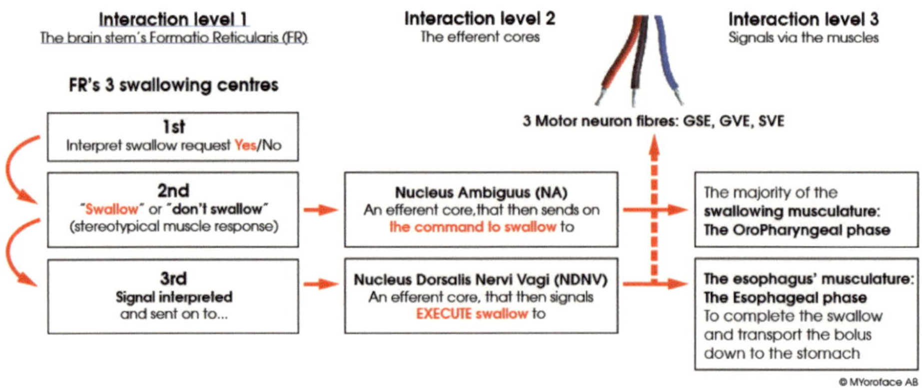

Figure 9.
The sensory-motoric reflex arc (level 1–3).

The 3rd swallowing center transmits information to the Nucleus Dorsalis Nervi Vagi (NDNV), and then onwards to the smooth muscles including those in the esophagus (**Figures 9** and **10**).

4.4 The motor neurons

The motor signals are transmitted via efferent nerves that can be thought of as cables containing various fibers and motor neurons to the muscles and glands. There are three different kinds of motor neurons that are important in the swallowing process (**Figure 10**) [5, 25, 29].

- The General Somatic Efferent (GSE) motor neurons are present in the CN Hypoglossus (XII) and CN Oculomotorius (III) which transmit signals onwards to the tongue's and the inner eyes' voluntary skeletal striated musculature.

- The Special Visceral Efferent (SVE) motor neurons act through the CN Trigeminus (V), CN Facialis (VII), CN Glossopharyngeus (IX), CN Vagus (X) and CN Accessorius (XI) which transmit signals to the voluntary musculature in the mouth, chewing muscles, facial musculature, pharynx, larynx, esophagus, and diaphragm.

- The General Visceral Efferent (GVE) motor neurons act via CN Facialis (VII) and CN Glossopharyngeus (IX) which transmit signals to the glands, blood vessels, and smooth muscles in the pharynx, stomach, and rectum.

The sum of all the above signals executes pre-programmed cooperation between the 148 muscles that are involved in the transport of each food bite from the mouth down to the stomach.

Motor neuron fibres	Cranial nerves	Muscles and glands
General Somatic Efferent (GSE) STRIATED MUSCULATURE 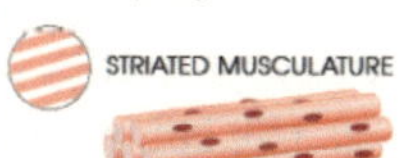	XII Hypoglossus III Oculomotorius	Tongue Eyes' inner muscles
Special Visceral Efferent (SVE) STRIATED MUSCULATURE 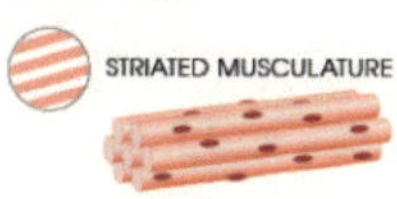	V Trigeminus m. tensor tympani VII Facialis m. stapedius IX Glossopharyngeus X Vagus XI Accessorius	Face Oral cavity Chewing muscles Eyes' outer muscles Pharynx Larynx Esophagus Diaphragm
General Visceral Efferent (GVE) SMOOTH MUSCULATURE 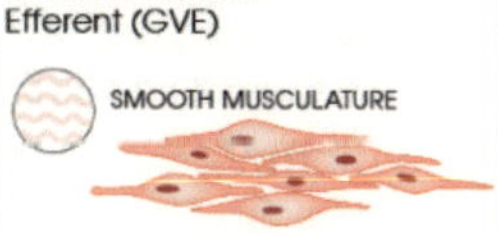	VII Facialis IX Glossopharyngeus	Glands Blood vessels Smooth musculature

Figure 10.
Three types of motor neurons.

The efferent nerves send signals via the three different motor neuron fiber types to the muscles and glands.

4.5 Understanding the three neurological phases

4.5.1 Oral phase

As we have said earlier, the oral phase is consciously controlled (voluntary) and is managed by the brain's cortex region [5, 25]. But when the bolus has passed the anterior palatal arch towards the pharynx, the swallow reflex takes over and this is controlled by the brain stem – no longer consciously or voluntarily controlled.

4.5.2 Pharyngeal phase

The tongue's movement backward and upwards transports the food towards the pharynx. When the bolus reaches the anterior palatal arch and the smooth palate, the reflexive phase of the swallow starts [5, 6] causing the larynx to rise, As the tongue begins its return movement forward, the epiglottis seals the airway and the food passes into the pharynx. The pharyngeal phase takes between 0.5 and 1 second.

In this phase, the coordination between breathing and swallowing is crucial to avoid food 'going down the wrong way' [5, 25, 30, 31]. Breathing and swallowing are guided by different centers in the brain stem, however, all the muscles that are active in these two functions are controlled from the same concentrated grouping of specialized nerves nucleus in the brain stem. This allows the swallowing center to take control of breathing during a crucial phase in the act of swallowing. When the 1st and 2nd Swallowing Centers signal that swallowing is underway, the body breathes in. During the subsequent exhalation, the food portion is driven to the back of the tongue and the exhalation stops as the bolus crosses the airway. Breathing ceases for 2 seconds about twice as long as it takes for the bolus to pass the pharynx then breathing is resumed with a continued exhalation.

4.5.3 Esophageal phase

The esophagus' longitudinal musculature forms a stiff pipe, the UES relaxes and opens to allow the passage of the bolus into the esophagus. The sphincter to the stomach – LES - opens to enable the entrance of the food.

The muscle function and the downwards transport of the bolus are controlled by the Vagus CN X and a branch of the Glossopharyngeal CN IX. Together these nerve pathways build a local network in the esophagus' *Plexus Pharyngeus* [25].

Both types of muscle: voluntary skeletal striated muscles and involuntary smooth muscles are present in the esophagus. The voluntary musculature is the same type as we have, for example, in our arms and legs: so-called skeletal striated muscles which are attached to the skeleton or tissue, and that are voluntarily controlled. The smooth musculature cannot be controlled voluntarily but is instead controlled by the autonomic nervous system: functioning unconsciously and involuntarily. These muscles are stimulated via the GVE motor neurons (**Figure 10**) in the brain stem which sends signals to the involuntary musculature.

The esophagus' upper third consists of skeletal striated muscles, the middle third is a mixture of skeletal striated muscles and smooth musculature, and the bottom third is solely smooth muscle.

5. Dysphagia and reflux diseases are related

5.1 What are reflux-based diseases?

This chapter has so far focussed mostly on the swallowing process of conveying food and drink to the stomach successfully, Hiatus hernia has been mentioned only in passing. Here we explain more about this condition. IQoro treats all dysfunctions in the process of swallowing food and drinks safely and successfully, and in retaining it in the stomach without reflux [14, 32]. A distinction between these two areas although often regarded as separate from a healthcare perspective is artificial. The same neuro-physiological processes are common to both dysfunctional swallowing and reflux.

5.1.1 Prevalence and symptoms

Reflux-based diseases are thought to affect around 20% of the world's population [33, 34]. Reflux is a condition in which stomach acids sometimes bubble up from the stomach, through the esophagus, and into the throat, larynx, and pharynx. The effect of these acids is to cause the symptoms of [35]:

- Heartburn
- Burning sensation in the chest
- Acidic reflux
- Swallowing difficulties
- Feeling of a lump in the throat
- Feeling of a blockage in the chest when eating
- Chest pains
- Pain under the breastbone (sternum)
- Stomach pains before eating
- Stomach pains after eating
- Reduced appetite
- Early "Full up" feeling
- Feeling sick
- Constipated, gassy
- Vomiting
- Persistent dry or phlegmy cough
- Food or drink 'goes down the wrong way'

- Hoarseness
- Breathing difficulties

It should be noted that if some of the above symptoms are chronic, and especially if they do not respond to medication, they could be caused by cancer or other diseases [36], and this should be considered before diagnosing reflux as the sole cause.

Refluxing stomach acids is the underlying cause of several conditions: LPR, GERD (or GORD), Silent Reflux, IED, Dyspepsia, etc. These conditions are sometimes known by their full names: Laryngopharyngeal Reflux, Gastroesophageal Reflux Disease, and Intermittent Esophageal Dysphagia. These various conditions exhibit some or all of the symptoms listed above, they vary slightly but are all caused by the corrosive effect of the refluxed stomach acids.

5.1.2 Cause of reflux

These symptoms occur when stomach acids reflux into the esophagus. The normal position of the stomach and the LES - the valve at the mouth of the stomach - is below the diaphragm. The esophagus passes through the diaphragm muscle through an aperture called the hiatus canal. In functional anatomy the muscle grips tightly around the esophagus and holds the stomach down in its correct position. The LES behaves like a trapdoor in this position, swinging downwards to let food and drink into the stomach before closing again. The LES cannot open upwards to allow reflux. An exception to this is if we need to belch or vomit; then the LES intrudes through the diaphragm slightly into the chest cavity and can flap open upwards and allow stomach gases, liquids or solids to reflux.

A Hiatal hernia is a weakening in the muscle that grips around the esophagus where it passes through the diaphragm. When this occurs the mouth of the stomach and the LES can intrude in an unwanted and uncontrolled fashion and allow reflux to occur.

5.1.3 Existing treatments for reflux-based diseases

The treatment options for reflux-based diseases fall into two broad camps: reducing the symptoms, or addressing the underlying cause.

In the former category, symptom reduction can be achieved by lifestyle changes or medication. Changing poor living, smoking, drinking, eating and diet habits can improve the impact of reflux, but lifestyle changes have an inconclusive effect [37].

Many Over the Counter (OTC) medications have a base pH and address the problem of reflux by reducing the acidity of the stomach acids which are being refluxed. Although the unpleasant sensations of reflux are reduced, the harmful effects on the vulnerable esophagus and other organs continue. Long-term use of OTC medication is generally regarded to be free from harmful side effects.

Prescribed PPI medications act by inhibiting the amount and strength of the acids produced in the stomach. PPI medications have significant known side effects and hence long-term PPI usage is generally discouraged and several countries insist that clinicians perform a medication review before renewing PPI prescriptions. At least once per year is recommended in the UK [38]. PPI medication is usually not expensive in itself, but the costs of repeat Healthcare Professional (HCP) interventions build to a considerable amount when prescribed for rest-of-life.

PPI drugs belong to one of the safest medication groups, but some research suggests a list of unwanted side effects [39, 40] include increased risk of cardiovascular disease, osteoporosis, dementia, male infertility, diabetes, and increased vulnerability to severe covid19 infection.

In addition, harmful bacteria in the stomach like Helicobacter pylori (HP) that would not survive in normal circumstances, can thrive in the weakened acids after PPI treatment. These germs can enter the body and live in the digestive tract. After many years, they can cause sores, called ulcers, in the lining of the stomach or the upper part of the small intestine. For some people, an infection can lead to stomach cancer.

In the case of all medications, there is no expectation that the underlying cause of the reflux – the weakened diaphragm musculature [34, 41]– will be addressed, merely the severity of the reflux symptoms.

The muscular deficiency at the root of the problem can sometimes be remedied by a surgical operation [42] that re-wraps muscles in the hiatal canal around the esophagus, or a similar procedure. Clearly, addressing the underlying cause is preferable in many ways to long-term medication and IQoro, as presented here, offers a simple non-invasive alternative to a surgical operation.

5.1.4 Existing treatments for dysphagia

As discussed, patients with a dysfunctional swallow sometimes after stroke are often treated with compensatory treatments [5, 6]. These care pathways allow patients to live within the limitations of their conditions. Direct and successful treatment of the dysfunctional swallowing chain is to be preferred and is presented in this chapter.

5.1.5 Treating the muscles

If the cause of both dysphagia and reflux is known to be neuromuscular, why are the most common treatments medication or surgical intervention? It is easy to grasp the idea that rebuilding muscle strength will improve swallowing, and allow the muscles in the Hiatal canal to regain their ability to grip around the esophagus.

If a patient presented with an arm that had atrophied because it had been in a plaster cast for some weeks, we might expect a rehab program based on weights and exercises. However, the atrophied-arm parallel has an important disconnect. As we have explained earlier, there are key differences between the arm muscles and many of the muscles that are needed to ensure an effective swallow and to prevent LES intrusion through the diaphragm allowing reflux. The arm is made up of skeletally striated muscles that can be commanded by the individual to flex, and can therefore be consciously exercised; whereas most of the muscles in the swallowing chain cannot, they are controlled and commanded through other nerve types and command systems. The paradox then is how to exercise muscles that cannot be commanded to flex.

6. IQoro

6.1 What is IQoro?

IQoro (**Figure 1**) is a simple hand-held plastic device that is inserted predentally (inside the lips and in front of the teeth) by a patient and pulled forward against lip pressure to exercise the swallow. At the time of writing, July 2021, it has been used by more than 50,000 individuals and is used by healthcare professionals to treat patients in hospitals and other settings across several countries. It is a CE-marked Class 1 Medical device, internationally patented and costing around USD 150.

6.2 How to train

The patient inserts the device pre-dentally and seals the lips against the handle, then pulls forward firmly displacing the lips forward slightly. This position is held for 10 seconds, followed by a short pause to relax, and then the action is repeated twice more. This 30-second training session should be carried out three times per day, preferably before mealtimes (**Figures 11–13**).

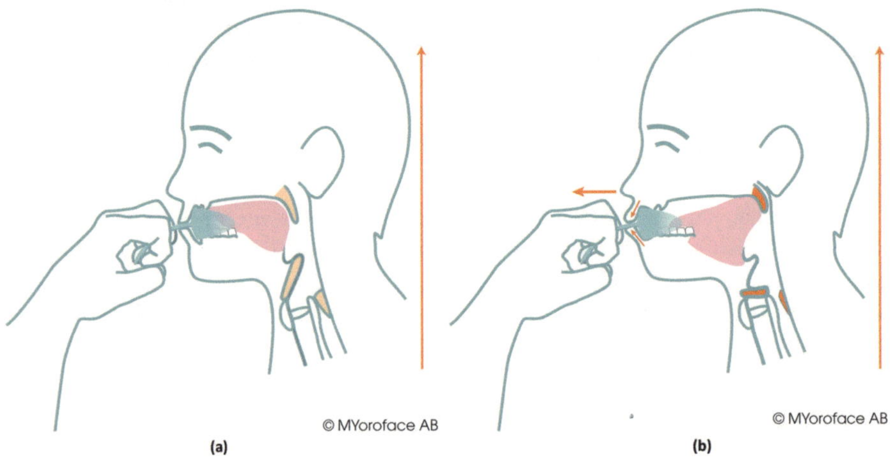

Figure 11.
(a, b): IQoro training action. (a) the IQoro is inserted pre-dentally, behind closed lips. (b) the patient presses his lips firmly together whilst pulling straight forward strongly for 5–10 seconds, and does this 3 times with 3 seconds rest between each pull. These sessions are performed three times per day, preferably before mealtimes. ***Video 1.***

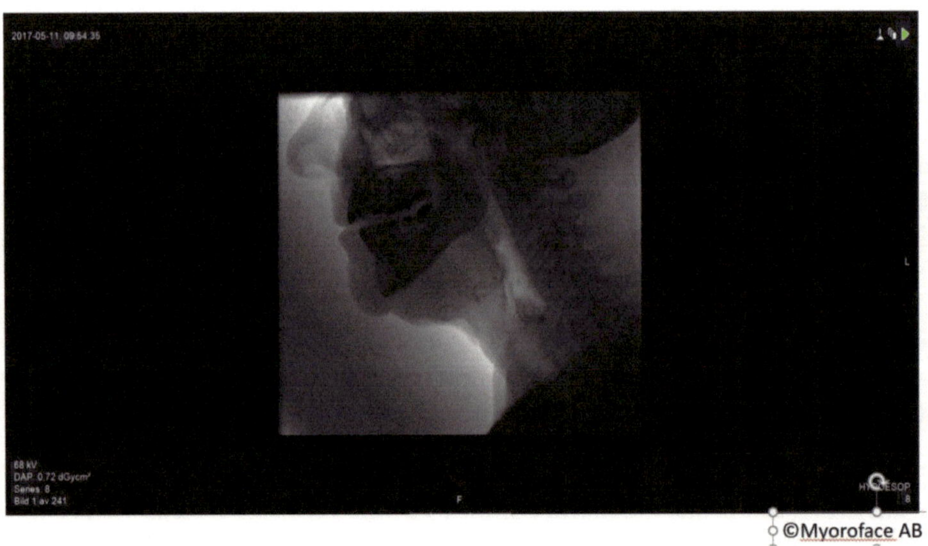

Figure 12.
Video 1. [43].

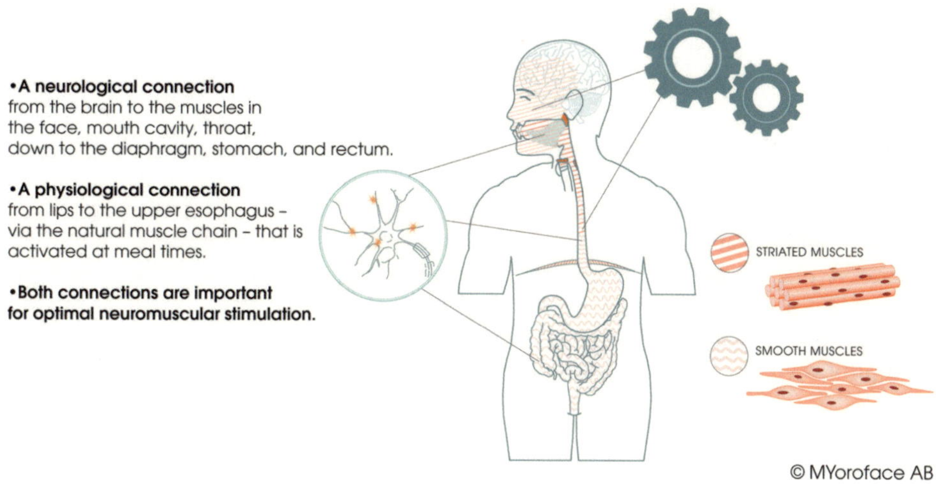

Figure 13.
Neurological and physiological considerations in muscle stimulation when eating or during neuromuscular training with IQoro.

Where a patient initially lacks lip strength or has diminished hand or arm function – perhaps after stroke - an assistant can help with this procedure. The vast majority of IQoro users self-treat without assistance.

6.3 How it works

IQoro causes all the muscles in the swallowing chain to be flexed and thus retrained and strengthened.

Training with IQoro triggers the sensory-motor reflex arc.

The muscles in the chain from the lips through to the upper third of the esophagus are mostly skeletally striated and are voluntarily activated [5, 29] when eating normally. Smooth musculature is present in the lower part of the esophagus, and down through the hiatus canal, LES, stomach, intestines, and rectum, and these muscles can only be activated by signals from the autonomic system [5, 29]. It is thus the case that striated musculature is activated by voluntary neurological and physiological commands, but the smooth muscle can only be activated and exercised via commands from the autonomic system.

Studies show that rehabilitation of the smooth musculature traditionally takes longer [14, 32, 44] and requires ongoing maintenance training after treatment.

When you close your lips tightly against the handle and pull the device forward, a low pressure is created in the mouth, making the tongue retract and seal against the anterior palatal arch and the soft palate. The effect of this is to strongly stimulate the sensory nerves in the oral cavity which send afferent signals to the brainstem as described in the neurology section above. Here they provoke a so-called sensory-motor reflex arc which causes intense efferent motor signals to exercise the muscles in the swallowing chain. In this way, IQoro training reaches and strengthens even the smooth musculature that cannot be voluntarily commanded by the patient.

Training with IQoro activates all the muscles in the swallowing chain, including the outer longitudinal muscles that run along the sides of the esophagus and fasten under the diaphragm. As they are activated by IQoro training they exercise the muscles at the site of the rupture, strengthening the weakened muscles back into a functional condition.

In other words, the training action and regime used to treat dysphagia [10] are equally appropriate for Hiatal hernia and reflux-based conditions [14, 32, 44].

7. Evidence of IQoro's efficacy

This section presents the scientific support for the efficacy of IQoro in treating the two closely related conditions of dysphagia and reflux-based diseases caused by a hiatal hernia. For reasons of space and readability, most studies have been reduced to short summaries of their purpose and conclusions and a link to the full article. Exceptions to this are 8.1.4 and 8.1.5 which are presented in more detail, having not been published in a scientific journal previously.

7.1 Dysphagia

7.1.1 Dysphagia studies

The evidence behind the efficacy of IQoro as a treatment for dysphagia includes more than a dozen peer-reviewed and internationally published scientific research papers.

7.1.1.1 Study: Effects on facial dysfunction and swallowing capacity of intraoral stimulation early and late after stroke

Study type

Peer-reviewed, prospective, cohort pre and post-study designed according to Good Clinical Practice (GCP) [15].

This study showed that IQoro is effective in improving swallowing ability, facial activity in all four facial quadrants in patients, and pharyngeal sling force after stroke, irrespective of time from stroke debut to start of treatment. Improvements were still present at late follow-up (>1 year after the end of treatment).

The 31 patients were grouped according to having had a stroke with recent onset, or a long time before. By implication, the similarly successful results in the two groups rule out spontaneous recovery as a likely cause of the improvements seen.

Conclusion

IQoro is effective in improving swallowing ability, facial activity in all four facial quadrants, and pharyngeal sling force after stroke, irrespective of time from stroke debut to start of treatment.

7.1.1.2 Study: Effect of IQoro training on impaired postural control and oropharyngeal motor function in patients with dysphagia after stroke

Study type

Peer-reviewed, prospective, cohort pre and post-study [17].

The study used IQoro as a treatment for 12 weeks in a patient group that had pathological levels for both Impaired Postural Control (IPC) and Oropharyngeal Motor Dysfunction (OPMD).

The 26 adults recruited to the study were divided between those with recent stroke, and those who had stroke onset a long time before. Results were equally positive in both groups showing the efficacy of IQoro in immediate intervention or in chronic sufferers. Once again, the similar results in the two groups rule out spontaneous recovery as a likely cause of the improvements seen.

At end of training significant improvement ($p < 0.001$) in tongue and velum function, velopharyngeal closure, and swallowing ability were recorded in the late intervention group. Almost all other outcome improvements in this group showed a ($p < 0.01$) statistical significance, as did all measures in the early intervention group.

Improvements were maintained at late follow-up (median 59 weeks after the end of training).

Two patients showed no improvement in either IPC or OPMD, all others regained normal abilities in both functions. Five patients presented with Percutaneous Endoscopic Gastrostomy (PEG) feeds at recruitment; all five PEGs were removed by/at end-of-training and all recovered the ability to eat and drink unmodified foods and liquids.

Conclusion

- IQoro successfully treats impaired postural control and oropharyngeal motor function in patients with dysphagia after stroke.
- PEGs can be removed after several years of use, after 3 months' IQoro treatment.
- Velum function is significantly improved by IQoro training.
- Improvements made are still present at long-term follow-up.
- The similarity of results in the two intervention groups further supports the contention that improvement is not due to spontaneous remission.
- The effectiveness of IQoro treatment is not affected by the time from stroke to the start of treatment, nor the age or gender of the patient.

The positive effect on muscle groups not directly accessed by IQoro neuromuscular training supports the contention that the improvements are triggered by neurological rehabilitation.

7.1.1.3 Study: Effects of oral neuromuscular training on swallowing dysfunction among older people in intermediate care: A cluster randomized, controlled trial

Study type

Peer-reviewed, prospective, cohort pre and post-study, Randomized Controlled Trial (RCT) [12].

385 elderly participants in intermediate care units were screened, and 116 with impaired swallowing were randomly assigned to IQoro neuromuscular training or usual care. Standard IQoro training was employed: 3 x 10 seconds, three times per day for 5 weeks and patients, were measured at three-time points: before training, at end of training, and at late follow up (6 months post-treatment).

- At end of treatment, the geometric mean of the swallowing rate in the intervention group had significantly improved 60% more than that of controls ($p = 0.007$).
- Signs of aspiration were significantly reduced in the intervention group compared with controls ($p = 0.01$).

- At 6 months post-treatment, the swallowing rate of the intervention group remained significantly better ($p = 0.031$).
- No significant between-group differences were found for swallowing-related quality of life.

Conclusion

Treatment ended at discharge from the residential facility in order that a long-term follow-up could determine that the improvements seen at end-of-treatment were sustained. Oral neuromuscular training is a new promising swallowing rehabilitation method for older people in intermediate care. Better clinical results would likely have been achieved if IQoro treatment had continued for longer than 5 weeks.

7.1.1.4 Study: Measuring the effectiveness of IQoro® treatment of saliva control dysfunction in children and young people with cerebral palsy using practice-based evidence outcome measures

This study is that performed by Natalie Morris and her team and referred to at the beginning of this chapter.

Saliva control difficulties.

Difficulty in controlling saliva is a common problem for people with Cerebral Palsy (CP). Drooling is not normally a result of overproduction but inefficient control of salivary secretions due to:

- Inadequate lip closure / habitual open mouth posture
- Reduced or impaired sensory feedback
- Atypical muscle tone
- Underlying swallowing difficulties
- Dental problems
- Side effects from other medications
- Impaired postural control

Existing and recommended treatments

Natalie's own clinical observations and experiences of working with children and young people (CYP) with CP were that difficulty with saliva control is a persistent problem with no real effective treatment. The Cochrane review of interventions for drooling in children with cerebral palsy concludes, "*There is no clear consensus on which interventions are safe and effective in managing drooling in children with CP. There is insufficient evidence to inform clinical practice on interventions for drooling in children with CP*" [24].

The UK's National Institute for Health and Care Excellence (NICE) guidance [23] on the assessment and management of CP in under 25 s recommends clinicians assess factors that may affect drooling in children and young people with cerebral palsy, these include:

- Compensatory strategies and management of contributory factors such as positioning - Multi-Disciplinary Teams (MDT) working with Occupational Therapists (OT) and Physiotherapists to promote head control.

- Increasing awareness of saliva - behavioral approaches to prompt children to swallow more often and wipe their faces. However, many people with CP have reduced sensory feedback and are often unaware that their chin is wet. Furthermore, the physical action of wiping their own chin can be difficult.

- Oral-motor therapy - aims to target musculature that can be voluntarily trained to improve muscle strength, tonicity, and coordination. However, from a neurological point of view, it is important to consider that although some of our swallows are initiated during the conscious process of eating, drinking, and specific exercises, the majority are reflexive: swallowing away our saliva without conscious involvement. The autonomic nervous system is responsible for the overall control of salivation: these nerves are not under conscious control.

- Improving oral health - reducing reflux and maintaining good oral hygiene will reduce the bacterial load of saliva and reduce the risk of infection.

- Eliminating mouthing behaviors - some tools that are provided to improve oral skills e.g., chewy tubes for jaw stability, can precipitate difficulties with saliva control if used incorrectly and not as part of a structured program.

Most CYP with CP is given some form of medication to help with saliva control.

NICE produced guidelines in 2017 [23] on the treatment of drooling in children with CP.

The most common medications prescribed are:

- Oral Glycopyrronium Bromide

  NICE concludes there is moderate evidence for the effectiveness of this treatment and no evidence for the long-term safety. Side effects include dry mouth, vomiting, constipation, and thickening of secretions, which may increase the risk of respiratory infection and pneumonia. Many children are kept on this medication for years, at great cost to the NHS (NICE gives an average of GBP 320 per bottle, around GBP 430 for 28 days' treatment, approx. GBP 5160 per year).

- Hyocine patches + Trihexyphenidyl Hydrochloride

  Although commonly prescribed, at the time of publication (January 2017), neither medication had a UK marketing authorization for use in CYP under 18 for treatment of hypersalivation.

- Finally, if other treatment methods have been investigated, Botulinum Toxin injections into the salivary glands or surgery to remove the glands may be considered. Although these would obviously be highly aversive experiences and considered only as a last resort.

IQoro as a possible treatment

In 2018, Natalie attended the Association of Speech and Language Therapists in Independent Practice (ASLTIP) conference in London and came across IQoro neuromuscular training device that exercises and strengthens the muscles needed for feeding and swallowing by activating the nervous system to and from the brain. The manufacturers suggest that while traditional oral-motor therapy can target.

The musculature that can be voluntarily trained to improve muscle strength, tonicity, and coordination, it does not target the two-thirds of the swallowing

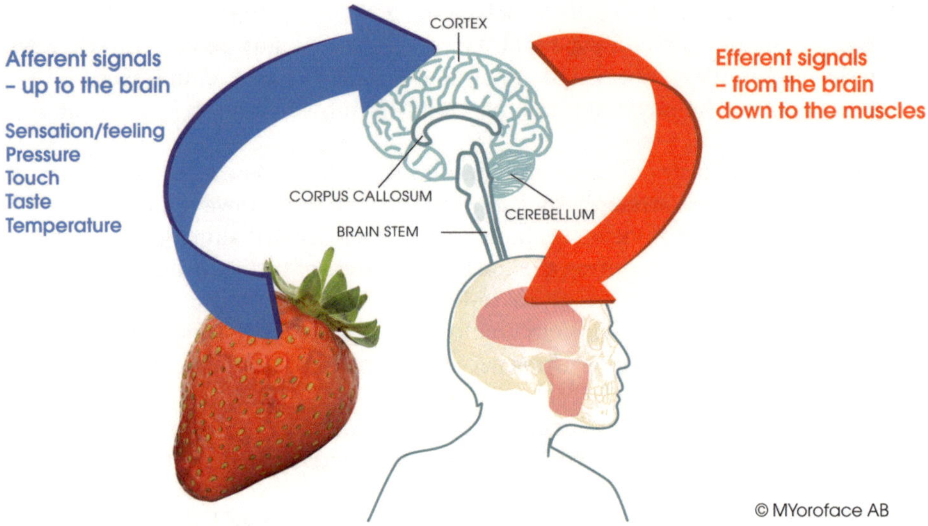

Figure 14.
The sensory-motoric reflex arc.

process that is controlled by the autonomic nervous system. IQoro claimed to trigger the sensory-motoric reflex arc which enables messages to be sent to musculature beyond the reach of voluntary control. The sensory-motoric reflex arc [5, 25], (**Figure 14**) effectively has a "leveraging" effect on direct muscular training and can improve the entire swallowing process.

IQoro could point to an impressive amount of research that had been conducted on adults with acquired swallowing difficulties, but no evidence to support its use with children. The question that interested Natalie was: "*Does IQoro improve saliva control in CYP with CP*?" Over a 20-week period, she collected ground-breaking practice-based evidence to answer this question.

Study method and design

The programme used a case series design: 10 participants aged between 6 and 22 years old all had a primary diagnosis of CP. A single case study design was applied to each individual and in addition to individual outcomes, inferences were drawn from the collective data.

Several measures were taken to establish baselines, and these were compared to the measurements taken after the treatment phase.

She and her team used a mixed-method strategy, producing quantitative data regarding oral motor and swallowing ability as well as collecting qualitative data about how the patients/carers / MDT members perceived the value of the tool.

Data collection & interventions

Natalie chose to use a Goal Attainment Scaling in Rehabilitation (GAS) method; GAS statistically scores the extent to which each patient's individual goals are achieved in the course of intervention. There is substantial literature that demonstrates its usefulness, both as part of the communication and decision-making process and as a person-centered outcome measure for rehabilitation [45]. Original: [46].

- Baseline assessments were taken of swallowing ability, oral motor function, and speech.
- Rating scales were used that allowed for skill breakdown and functional description of each area.

- The baseline assessment scores were used to set for intervention.
- An individual program for using the IQoro was designed for each patient and then carried out 3 x per day (by parents/carers) for 20 weeks.

Results

The composite GAS is transformed into a standardized measure with a mean of 50. If goals are set in an unbiased fashion, one would expect a normal distribution of scores, and the GAS thus performs at the interval level. If goals have been fully achieved, we would expect to see a score of 50 (**Table 1**).

Results indicated that IQoro does improve saliva control in children with CP, with improvements also demonstrated with oral motor skills. Using the measures of articulation, there was no change to speech. However, changes to voice were observed in the qualitative analysis (**Table 2**).

GAS Score	Swallowing	Oral Motor	Speech
Baseline	35.1	34.5	32.2
Range	34.9–35.8	31.3–36.3	26.5–35.2
Achieved	53.7	48.1	32.2
Range	44.3–60.3	45.8–51.6	26.5–35.2
Change	18.8	13.6	0
Range	8.5–25.3	10.6–20.3	0

Table 1.
Results showing GAS scores pre and post-treatment.

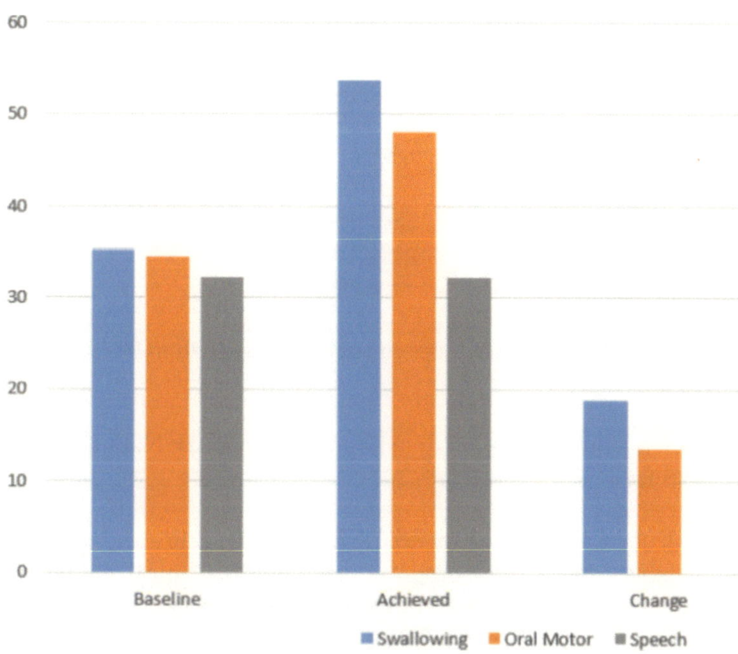

Table 2.
Improved outcomes in swallowing and oral motor skills, but not speech.

Discussion, quantitative and qualitative analysis

In this study, it has been possible to demonstrate an improvement with saliva control resulting from treatment using IQoro. On average, ratings reduced from 4 ("unable to control", saliva loss 75–100% of the time) to 2 ("moderate difficulty", saliva loss 25–50% of the time). However, at least half of the participants improved further to a score of 1 ("mild difficulty", saliva loss 10–25% of the time).

Qualitative data reported (but not measured) saw improvements with: teeth brushing; nasal breathing; breath control for speech; reduction in chest infections; sensory feedback (perception of saliva on chin) and tongue retraction. Positive feedback has been received from schools (less damage from saliva to IT equipment and worksheets) and physio colleagues (able to work in supine for longer periods due to an increase in swallowing of secretions).

Future plans include creating an assessment protocol and running a training program. Further research is indicated to see if this would be a cost-effective treatment that could be made available on the NHS.

Conclusion

It has been the case that there is a severe lack of options in treating children and young people with Cerebral Palsy with dysfunction that leads to drooling. Existing medication and surgical intervention alternatives are often ineffective, invasive, and even not strictly approved for patients in these age groups. Many medication alternatives are expensive when compared with IQoro treatment.

IQoro has been proved to be a suitable treatment for the group studied, including those at the higher end of the scale of motoric and other difficulties. In the case of some of the latter, two assistants were required to perform the training.

Swallowing and oral motor competence improved significantly to a level around the 50-point target of the GAS goals, although the measured speech ability did not. Other functions and abilities important in daily life also improved as reported above.

Much-improved drooling and saliva control had great influence in improving the patients' quality of life, not least where it allowed the use of laptops, books, and other educational material in schools.

7.1.1.5 Study: IQoro dysphagia therapy in an NHS setting: A service evaluation

Roseanne, Exell 1; Hayley McBain 2; Sam Turvey 2; Gill Hardy 1

1. Royal Devon and Exeter NHS Foundation Trust

2. South West Academic Health Science Network

A service evaluation was carried out in southern England in 2020 resulting in the following abstract.

Background

This evaluation explored the introduction of IQoro into a National Health Service (NHS) setting.

Method

Patients with chronic dysphagia were recruited from acute and community settings and completed a 12-week program using IQoro. Clinical and well-being measures were taken pre and post-training. Feedback was gained from the Speech and Language Therapists delivering this program.

Results

25 patients were recruited into the evaluation, 21 completed the program. There were significant improvements in self-reported quality of life scores, including the

overall scores and burden of dysphagia and mental health subscales. There was a significant improvement in functional measures of dysphagia, including the consistencies of food and drink that patients could safely manage. There was also a significant improvement in the facial movement and symmetry of the lower half of the face. Feedback from SLTs indicated that IQoro improved the range of therapy options available and many planned to use it again. Qualitative feedback suggested that the use of IQoro may change SLTs clinical thinking, including in relation to intervention or compensation for dysphagia.

Conclusion

IQoro can be successfully introduced into an NHS team and can be effective in supporting patients with chronic dysphagia. However, factors such as the ability to follow patients across different settings and the individual risk of further decline need to be considered.

7.1.1.6 Customer survey

In an email survey in June 2021 of all IQoro users that had purchased within the previous 1–15 months, users were canvassed on the effectiveness of IQoro treatment for dysphagia. Totally 4440 responses were received, 983 were specifically treating symptoms associated with dysphagia after stroke. Patients had trained for 1 month or more (**Table 3**).

Conclusion

This survey of a large population of people using IQoro to treat various types of dysphagia and facial weakness is that their outcome experience is positive. This survey differs from the studies quoted elsewhere in this chapter in that the results shown are not at end-of-training in all cases. Many had not trained long enough at the time of the survey to experience the full effect in symptom reductions: some having only trained for as little as 1 month. Nevertheless, 79% - 86% reported symptom improvements since starting training.

7.1.1.7 Medtech Innovation Briefings

The UK's National Institution for Health and Care Excellence (NICE)), was commissioned by the UK government and advises and supports National Health Service and social care commissioners and have made a review of IQoro and its claims and effectiveness. They have issued a Medtech Innovation Briefing [47] that recognized "*IQoro is an innovative treatment, with no similar technologies currently recommended, and that the intended place in therapy would be in addition to standard speech and language therapy in people with stroke-related dysphagia*".

	Symptom free	Big improvement	Small improvement	No improvement yet	
Difficulty in swallowing liquids safely	11%	42%	33%	14%	100%
Difficulty in swallowing solid foods	7%	35%	38%	21%	100%
Drooling	9%	24%	44%	23%	100%
Facial or speech weakness	4%	28%	47%	21%	100%

Table 3.
Improved outcomes in swallowing and facial abilities.

7.1.2 Hiatus hernia and reflux-based conditions

Reflux occurs when the neck of the stomach and the Lower Esophageal Sphincter (LES) intrude through the diaphragm into the chest cavity. In this position, the LES can open upwards and allow stomach contents to reflux, in its correct position it can only allow one-way traffic downwards. This intrusion or hernia is made possible when the musculature of the diaphragm around the hiatal canal is weakened (**Figure 15**).

IQoro is an effective treatment for reflux-based diseases and their various symptoms: heartburn, pain behind the sternum, persistent unproductive cough, blockage in the throat, and more. Training with IQoro provokes stimuli from the brainstem to flex and strengthen all the muscles in the swallowing chain including those allowing a Hiatal hernia.

The evidence behind the efficacy of IQoro as a treatment for Hiatus hernia includes the following three peer-reviewed and internationally published scientific research papers which are briefly summarized here.

7.1.2.1 Study: Esophageal dysphagia and reflux symptoms before and after oral IQoro training

Study type

Peerreviewed, Prpospective, cohort pre and post-study [14].

43 patients who had esophageal dysphagia for a median of 3 years (range: 1–15 years) were recruited to this study. All displayed the symptoms of a Hiatal hernia, but only 21 had had their condition confirmed by examination. All had been prescribed Proton Pump Inhibitor (PPI) medication for more than 1 year without any effect, all medication ceased at the start of IQoro treatment.

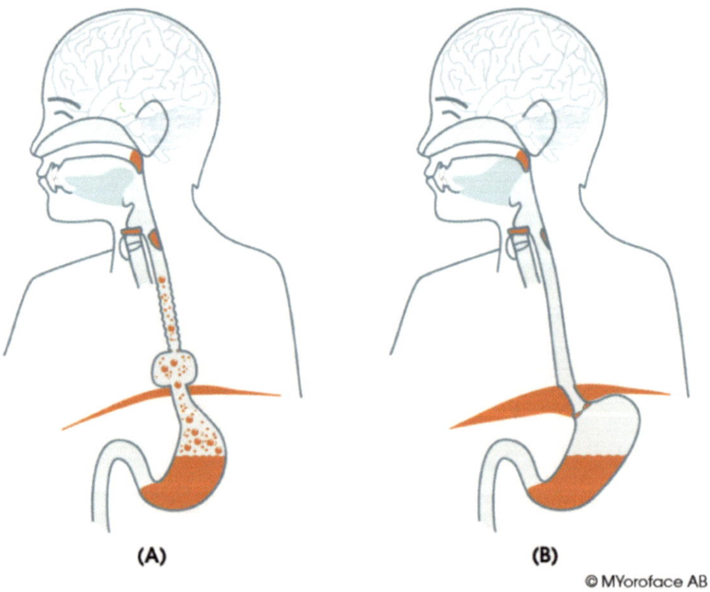

Figure 15.
(A) Sliding hiatal hernia. The upper part of the stomach and the LES has slid up through the hiatal canal. This allows gastroesophageal reflux and also causes difficulties with opening the PES at the top of the esophagus. (B) Normal anatomy. The neck of the stomach is correctly held below the diaphragm promoting normal LES function and preventing reflux.

Outcome measurements

A validated test battery was employed at baseline and at end of training including questionnaires and tests for all patients. In addition to these measures 12 patients with confirmed hiatal hernia were measured using High Resolution Manometry (HRM) [48] to measure pressure at resting and during IQoro traction.

Results

- No statistical difference (p = NS) between symptoms or outcomes between those with or without confirmed Hiatal hernia diagnosis – both before and after treatment.
- Esophageal dysphagia was present in all 43 patients at start of treatment, and 98% of patients showed improvement after IQoro neuromuscular training ($p < 0.001$).
- Reflux symptoms were reported before training in 86% of the patients, 100% of these showed improvement at end of training, ($p < 0.001$) and 58% were entirely symptom free. All patients ceased PPI medication at recruitment to the study.
- VAS scores were classified as pathologic in all 43 patients, and 100% showed improvement after IQoro neuromuscular training ($p < 0.001$).
- Pharyngeal sling force and velum closure test values were both significantly higher ($p < 0.001$) after IQoro neuromuscular training.

Those tested with HRM showed the following results:

- During IQoro traction there was an increase in mean pressure in the diaphragmatic hiatus region and in the Upper Esophageal Sphincter (UES) (**Table 4**).

Conclusion

IQoro neuromuscular training can relieve/improve esophageal dysphagia and reflux symptoms in adults, likely due to improved hiatal competence. The similarity of the results in the two groups suggests that many people suffer from Hiatus hernia despite this not having been confirmed by diagnosis.

7.1.2.2 Study: Effect of IQoro training in hiatal hernia patients with misdirected swallowing and esophageal retention symptoms

Study type

Peer-reviewed, prospective, cohort pre and post-study [17].

Items Pressures in mmHg	UES n = 12	Hiatus n = 12
Normal pressure	>30	10–35
Resting pressure	68 (40–110)	0 (0–0)
During IQoro traction	95 (80–130)	65 (20–100)

Data are mean (range) mmHg.

Table 4.
High-resolution manometry (HRM) results in UES and hiatus both at rest and during IQoro traction.

The study investigated whether 28 patients with hiatal hernia and misdirected swallowing and esophageal retention symptoms could be successfully treated with a 6-month regime of standard IQoro training: 30 seconds three times per day. Patients had had their condition for median of 4 years (range 1–28).

Results

- Reflux symptoms were reported before training in all patients,

  100% of these showed improvement ($p < 0.001$) at end of the training, and 61% were entirely symptom-free despite ceasing PPI medication at the start of training.

- All hiatal hernia patients were improved after training with IQoro and showed significant improvements ($p < 0.001$) in

  - misdirected swallowing,
  - cough,
  - hoarseness,
  - esophageal retention,
  - globus sensation,
  - scores for VAS, pharyngeal sling force, VCT, and TWST.

- Traction during the training action with IQoro resulted in a 65 mmHg increase in the mean pressure of the diaphragmatic hiatus as measured by high-resolution manometry (**Table 4**).

Conclusion

IQoro training significantly improves all the symptoms of hiatus hernia, likely through improved hiatal competence.

7.1.2.3 Study: Oral neuromuscular training relieves hernia-related dysphagia and GERD symptoms as effectively in obese as in non-obese patients

Study type

Peer reviewed, prospective, clinical study, cohort pre and post-study [32].

It has been thought that treatment of Hiatus hernia in overweight patients can be unproductive and that weight loss should be a prior step to interventions.

In this study 86 adult patients with verified hiatal hernias and long-standing Intermittent Esophageal Disease (IED) and other Gastro-Esophageal Reflux Disease (GERD) symptoms were grouped according to their Body Mass Index (BMI), before entry into the study (**Table 5**): Group A: normal weight, Group B: moderately obese, Group C: severely obese.

Results

At entry into the study there were no significant differences between the three BMI groups in baseline testing for swallowing ability, or for IED and GERD symptom severity, except that:

- Heartburn and cough were significantly more common in Groups B (moderately obese) and C (severely obese).

Items	Group A; *n* = 37	Group B; *n* = 28	Group C; *n* = 21
Median age	69 yrs. (20–85)	57 yrs. (22–85)	62 yrs. (44–87)
Gender	19 women, 18 men	16 women, 12 men	11 women, 10 men
GERD symptom duration	5 yrs. (1–75)	6 yrs. (1–15)	3 yrs. (1–29)
BMI before/after IQNT	23 (17–24) /23 (20–25)	28 (26–29) / 27 (24–29)	33 (30–37) / 31 (27–38)

Ranges in parentheses. BMI and GERD: median values; IQNT: Neuromuscular training with an oral IQoro.

Table 5.
Analysis of subjects by BMI grouping - age, gender, and GERD symptom duration.

- Misdirected swallowing was significantly more common in Group C.

After IQoro neuromuscular training, the following was observed in all three BMI groups:

- All IED and GERD symptom scores were significantly improved or reduced ($p < 0.001$).
- Median BMI was not significantly changed.
- Self-assessed GERD symptom improvement showed no significant difference across the groups, except for heartburn, cough, and misdirected swallowing which were significantly ($p < 0.01$) more reduced in obese patients than in normal bodyweight patients.
- The swallowing tests showed significant improvement ($p < 0.001$) in median values, with no significant difference between the BMI groups except for:
    - Timed Water Swallow Test (TWST) values, which were significantly ($p < 0.01$) more improved in Group C (severely obese) than in Group A (normal weight).
    - pharyngeal sling force, which was significantly ($p < 0.05$) more improved in Group B (moderately obese) than in Group A.

Conclusion

IQoro neuromuscular training (IQNT), a non-surgical treatment for IED and other GERD symptoms in hiatal hernia patients, is equally successful in treating moderately or severely obese patients as in treating sufferers of normal weight. Obesity in itself does not, therefore, seem to be a handicap in treating IED and other GERD symptoms by IQNT.

7.1.2.4 Customer survey

In an email survey in June 2021 of all IQoro users that had purchased within the previous 15 months, users were canvassed on the effectiveness of IQoro treatment for dysphagia. Totally 4440 responses were received of which 3436 were specifically treating classic reflux symptoms caused by Hiatus hernia, the rest of the responses were from people treating symptoms associated with dysphagia after stroke or snoring and sleep apnoea. Patients had trained for 1 month or more.

	Symptom free	Big improvement	Small improvement	No improvement yet	
Reflux / acid reflux	6%	40%	37%	17%	100%
Heartburn	9%	42%	34%	15%	100%
A sensation of something stuck in your throat	12%	38%	34%	17%	100%
Excessive or thick phlegm	4%	30%	42%	24%	100%
Dry, persistent cough	8%	34%	36%	22%	100%
Gassy, burping often	4%	35%	39%	22%	100%
Pain in your chest or esophagus	11%	39%	33%	17%	100%
Food that you have swallowed comes up again	15%	38%	31%	16%	100%
Hoarseness	8%	29%	39%	24%	100%

Table 6.
Improved outcomes in hiatal hernia related symptoms.

76%–84% of respondents reported symptom improvement, it can be assumed that some of those not yet reporting improvements had only trained for a short while (**Table 6**).

Conclusion

A large population, 3436 people, using IQoro to treat reflux symptoms showed positive outcome experiences. This survey differs from the studies quoted elsewhere in this chapter in that the results shown are not at end-of-training in all cases. Many had not trained long enough at the time of the survey to experience the full effect in symptom reductions: some having only trained for as little as 1 month. Nevertheless, 76% - 85% reported symptom improvements since starting training.

7.1.3 NICE Medtech innovation briefing

In March 2019 the UK's National Institute for Health and Care Excellence (NICE) developed a Medtech Innovation Briefing (MIB) [49] regarding the use of IQoro to treat Hiatus hernia, it points out the innovative nature of the device and its potential to save the NHS money.

> *"The NICE MIB highlights the innovative nature of IQoro as being its uniqueness in treating Hiatus Hernia through an exercise regime with an oral device. It also highlights that the resource impact of using IQoro could be to reduce costs for the NHS in the long term, one of the main points of our analysis of possible cost savings in this briefing is the device's potential to be resource releasing when compared to long term PPI maintenance."*

8. Conclusions

All versions of dysphagia have an unsatisfactory range of treatment options. Swallowing difficulties, reflux, and other manifestations are often met with compensatory strategies instead of the treatment of the underlying causes. IQoro is simple, inexpensive, non-invasive, and takes just 90 seconds per day.

IQoro is proven both in clinical practice and in research studies to be highly effective in treating the underlying causes of the conditions and symptoms described in this book. The evidence base for its efficacy is strong.

This innovative device and treatment are shown to be effective in treating all types of dysphagia in the pre-oral, oral, pharyngeal, and esophageal phases. Similarly, Hiatus hernia and its resulting reflux symptoms can be addressed successfully. In all of these conditions, it is shown that time from onset of the condition stroke or Hiatus hernia for example, to the time when IQoro treatment starts, does not affect the positive outcome results of the treatment. The stroke studies show that improvements achieved at end-of-treatment persist at long-term follow-up. Several studies and evaluations show that patients with PEG feeding tubes have had them removed after IQoro therapy.

All healthcare professionals working with dysphagia and its related conditions should want to know more about IQoro and how it improves patient outcomes and gives clinicians an important and powerful new treatment option.

Acknowledgements

The authors would like to thank Terry Morris (no relation to the author) for his assistance in authoring this chapter, for creating the summary of abstracts from which several of the above studies are copied, and for performing the data analysis on the customer survey referred to above.

The authors would also like to thank Gill Hardy, Speech and Language Therapist, Clinical Lead Neurology, and her colleagues at the Royal Devon and Exeter NHS Foundation Trust and also Roseanne Exell and Hayley McBain at the South West Academic Health Science Network for their kind permission to reproduce the abstract of their service evaluation shown above.

Some studies reproduced above were supported by grants from The Centre for Research & Development, Uppsala University/County Council of Gävleborg, Gävle, Sweden, and The Council for Regional Research in Uppsala and Örebro region, Sweden.

Conflict of interest

IQoro is patented in Sweden - SE 1350314-9, 2014 July 14 - and widely internationally. It is CE-marked as a Class 1 Medical Device for therapeutic use by the manufacturer MYoroface AB. Mary Hägg is the inventor.

The authors, Mary Hägg and Natalie Morris declare that they have no conflict of interest.

Notes/thanks/other declarations

All studies were performed according to the Helsinki Declaration. Informed written and verbal consent was obtained from all the participants in the studies. All images are kindly provided by MYoroface AB.

Author details

Mary Hägg[1,2]* and Natalie R. Morris[3,4,5]

1 Assoc. Prof., DDS. Speech and Swallowing Centre, Department of Otorhinolaryngology, Hudiksvall Hospital, Hudiksvall, Sweden

2 Centre for Research and Development, Uppsala University/Region, Gävleborg, Sweden

3 Reg. Mem. RCSLT, HCPC

4 The Feeding Trust, Birmingham, UK. (Founder and CEO)

5 Integrated Therapy Solutions, Birmingham, UK. (Clinical Lead)

*Address all correspondence to: mary@myoroface.com

References

[1] Serra-Prat M, Palomera M, Gomez C, Sar-Shalom D, Saiz A, Montoya JG, et al. Oropharyngeal dysphagia as a risk factor for malnutrition and lower respiratory tract infection in independently living older persons: A population-based prospective study. Age and Ageing. 2012;**41**(3): 376-381

[2] Martino R, Foley N, Bhogal S, Diamant N, Speechley M, Teasell R. Dysphagia after stroke: Incidence, diagnosis, and pulmonary complications. Stroke. 2005;**36**(12): 2756-2763

[3] Ekberg O, Hamdy S, Woisard V, Wuttge-Hannig A, Ortega P. Social and psychological burden of dysphagia: Its impact on diagnosis and treatment. Dysphagia. 2002;**17**(2):139-146

[4] Neyens J, Halfens R, Spreeuwenberg M, Meijers J, Luiking Y, Verlaan G, et al. Malnutrition is associated with an increased risk of falls and impaired activity in elderly patients in Dutch residential long-term care (LTC): A cross-sectional study. Archives of Gerontology and Geriatrics. 2013; **56**(1):265-269

[5] Logemann JA. Evaluation and Treatment of Swallowing Disorders. 2nd ed. Austin, Tex: PRO-ED; 1998

[6] Ekberg O, Hamdy S, Woisard V, Wuttge-Hannig A, Ortega P. Social and psychological burden of dysphagia: Its impact on diagnosis and treatment. Dysphagia. 2002;**17**:139-146. DOI: 10.1007/s00455-001-0113-5

[7] Shaker R, Easterling C, Kern M, et al. Rehabilitation of swallowing by exercise in tube-fed patients with pharyngeal dysphagia secondary to abnormal UES opening. Gastroenterology. 2002;**122**: 1314-1321. DOI: 10.1053/gast.2002.32999

[8] Huckabee ML, Cannito MP. Outcomes of swallowing rehabilitation in chronic brainstem dysphagia: A retrospective evaluation. Dysphagia. 1999;**14**:93-109

[9] Crary MA, Carnaby GD, LaGorio LA, Carvajal PJ. Functional and physiological outcomes from an exercisebased dysphagia therapy: A pilot investigation of the McNeill Dysphagia Therapy Program. Archives of Physical Medicine and Rehabilitation. 2012;**93**: 1173-1178. DOI: 10.1016/j.apmr.2011.11.008

[10] Hägg M, Anniko M. Lip muscle training in stroke patients with dysphagia. Acta Oto-Laryngologica. 2008;**128**(9):1027-1033

[11] Hägg M, Tibbling L. Longstanding effect and outcome differences of palatal plate and oral screen training on stroke related dysphagia. The Open Rehabilitation Journal. 2013;**6**: 35-42

[12] Hagglund P, Hagg M, Wester P, Levring JE. Effects of oral neuromuscular training on swallowing dysfunction among older people in intermediate care-a cluster randomised, controlled trial. Age and Ageing. 2019; **48**(4):533-540

[13] Hagg M, Anniko M. Influence of lip force on swallowing capacity in stroke patients and in healthy subjects. Acta Oto-Laryngologica. 2010;**130**(11): 1204-1208

[14] Hägg M, Tibbling L, Franzén T. Esophageal dysphagia and reflux symptoms before and after oral IQoro® training. World Journal of Gastroenterology. 2015;**21**(24): 7558-7562. Open access: http://www.wjgnet.com/1007- 9327/full/v21/i24/7558.htm

[15] Hägg MK, Tibbling LI. Effects on facial dysfunction and swallowing capacity of intraoral stimulation early and late after stroke. NeuroRehabilitation. 2015;**36**(1): 101-106. DOI: 10.3233/NRE-141197 PMID: 25547771

[16] Hagg M, Tibbling L. Effect of oral IQoro® and palatal plate training in post-stroke, four-quadrant facial dysfunction and dysphagia: A comparison study. Acta Oto-Laryngologica. 2015;**135**:962-968. DOI: 10.3109/00016489.2015.1042043

[17] Hägg M, Tibbling L. Effect of IQoro® training on impaired postural control and oropharyngeal motor function in patients with dysphagia after stroke. Acta Oto-Laryngologica. 2016;**136**(7):742-748. DOI: 10.3109/00016489.2016.1145797

[18] Hägg M, Olgarsson M, Anniko M. Reliable lip force measurement in healthy controls and in patients with stroke. A methodological study. Dysphagia. 2008;**2**:291-296

[19] Perkins RE, Blanton PL, Biggs N. Electromyographic analysis of the "buccinator mechanism" in human beings. Journal of Dental Research. 1977; **56**:783-794

[20] Hägg M, Larsson B. Effects of motor and sensory stimulation in stroke patients with long-lasting dysphagia. Dysphagia. 2004;**19**:219-230

[21] Ney DM, Weiss JM, Kind AJH, Robbins J. Senescent Swallowing: Impact, Strategies, and Interventions. Nutrition in Clinical Practice. 2009; **24**(3):395-413

[22] Carnaby G, Hankey GJ, Pizzi J. Behavioural intervention for dysphagia in acute stroke: a randomised controlled trial. Lancet Neurology. 2006 Jan;**5**(1): 31-37

[23] Severe sialorrhoea (drooling) in children and young people with chronic neurological disorders: Oral glycopyrronium bromide https://www.nice.org.uk/advice/es5/chapter/Introduction-and-current-guidance.x

[24] Walshe M, Smith M, Pennington L. Interventions for drooling in children with cerebral palsy. Cochrane Database of Systematic Reviews. 2012;**11**: CD008624. DOI: 10.1002/14651858.CD008624.pub3

[25] Ertekin C, Aydogdu I. Neurophysiology of swallowing. Clinical Neurophysiology. 2003;**114**:2226-2244

[26] Castillo Morales RC, Brondo JJ, Haberstock B. Die orofaziale Regulationstherapie. 1st ed. München: Richard Pflaum Verlag GmbH & Co.; 1991. pp. 21-188

[27] Ekberg O, Nylander G. Pharyngeal constrictor paresis in patients with dysphagia: A cineradiographic study. Clinical Radiology. 1982;**33**:253-258

[28] Ekberg O, Nylander G. Dysfunction of the cricopharyngeal muscle. A cineradiographic study of patients with dysphagia. Radiology. 1982;**143**:481-486

[29] Logemann JA. Screening, diagnosis and management of neurogenic dysphagia. Seminars in Neurology. 1996;**16**:319-327

[30] Preiksaitis HG, Mills CA. Coordination of breathing and swallowing: Effects of bolus consistency and presentation in normal adults. Journal of Applied Physiology. 1996;**81**: 1707-1714

[31] Smith J, Wolkove N, Colacone A, Kreisman H. Coordination of eating, drinking, and breathing in adults. Chest. 1989;**96**:578-582

[32] Franzén T, Tibbling L, Hägg M. Oral neuromuscular training relieves

hernia-related dysphagia and GERD symptoms as effectively in obese as in non-obese patients. Acta Oto-Laryngologica. 2018 Nov;**138**(11): 1004-1008. DOI: 10.1080/00016489.2018.1503715 Epub 2019 Jan 10

[33] Yu HX, Han CS, Xue JR, et al. Esophageal hiatal hernia: Risk, diagnosis and management. Expert Review of Gastroenterology & Hepatology. 2018; **12**(4):319-329

[34] Siegal SR, Dolan JP, Hunter JG. Modern diagnosis and treatment of hiatal hernias. Langenbeck's Archives of Surgery. 2017;**402**(8): 1145-1151

[35] Franzén T, Boström J, Tibbling Grahn L, et al. Prospective study of symptoms and gastro-oesophageal reflux 10 years after posterior partial fundoplication. The British Journal of Surgery. 1999;**86**:956-960. DOI: 10.1046/j.1365-2168.1999.01183.x

[36] Choueiri NE, Prather CM. Choueiri NE, et al. Barrett's esophagus: a pre-cancerous condition approach to diag nosis and management. Missouri Medicine 2009;**106**(5):339–342. PMID: 19902713

[37] Stein E, Sloan J, Sonu I, et al. GERD for the nongastroenterologist: Successful evaluation, management, and lifestyle-based symptom control. Annals of the New York Academy of Sciences. Dec 2020;**1482**(1):106-112. DOI: 10.1111/nyas.14496

[38] National Institute for Health and Care Excellence. Gastro-Oesophageal Reflux Disease and Dyspepsia in Adults: Investigation and Management. (September 2014) (CG184). Available at: www.nice.org.uk/guidance/cg184/resources/gastrooesophageal-reflux-disease-and-dyspepsia-inadults-investigation-and-management-35109812699845

[39] Bjornsson E, Abrahamsson H, Simren M, et al. Discontinuation of proton pump inhibitors in patients on long-term therapy: A double-blind, placebo-controlled trial. Alimentary Pharmacology & Therapeutics. 2006; **24**(6):945-954

[40] Chubineh S, Birk J. Proton pump inhibitors: The good, the bad, and the unwanted. Southern Medical Journal. 2012;**105**(11):613-618. DOI: 10.1097/SMJ.0b013e31826efbea

[41] Johansson KE, Ask P, Boeryd B, Fransson SG, Tibbling L. Oesophagitis, signs of reflux, and gastric acid secretion in patients with symptoms of gastrooesophageal reflux disease. Scandinavian Journal of Gastroenterology. 1986;**21**:837-847 [PMID: 3775250]

[42] Mayo D, Darbyshire A, Mercer S, et al. Technique and outcome of day case laparoscopic hiatus hernia surgery for small and large hernias: A five-year retrospective reflux as a risk factor for esophageal adenocarcinoma. The New England Journal of Medicine. 1999; **340**(11):825-831. Review from a high-volume UK centre. Ann R Coll Surg Engl. 2020 Oct;102(8):611–615. DOI: 10.1308/rcsann.2020.0151. Epub 2020 Jul 31

[43] Video 1_IQoro_This is how you exercise_A short version.

[44] Hägg M, Tibbling L, Franzén T. Effect of IQoro® training in hiatal hernia patients with misdirected swallowing and esophageal retention symptoms. Acta Oto-Laryngologica. 2015;**135**(7):635-639

[45] Hurn J, Kneebone I, Cropley M. Goal setting as an outcome measure: A systematic review. Clinical Rehabilitation. 2006;**20**(9):756-772

[46] Kiresuk T, Sherman R. Goal attainment scaling: A general method of

evaluating comprehensive mental health programmes. Community Mental Health Journal. 1968;**4**:443-453

[47] Medtech Innovation Briefing produced by the UK's National Institute for Health and Care Excellence in 2019. Available from: https://www.nice.org.uk/advice/mib175

[48] Tibbling L, Gezelius P, Franzén T. Factors influencing lower esophageal sphincter relaxation after deglutition. World Journal of Gastroenterology. 2011;**17**:2844-2847 [PMID: 21734792]. DOI: 10.3748/wjg.v17.i23.2844

[49] Medtech Innovation Briefing produced by the UK's National Institute for Health and Care Excellence in 2019. Available from: https://www.nice.org.uk/advice/mib176

Chapter 9

The Nutritional Challenges in Dysphagia: Not Only a Matter of Nutrients

Isabelle Germain

Abstract

Oropharyngeal dysphagia can significantly affect food ingestion. Texture-modified foods and thickened fluids are proposed to alleviate this difficulty. The nutritional density of adapted foods is often insufficient to maintain adequate nutritional intakes. The current scientific knowledge relies on a weak correlation between clinical assessment and meals consumed by patients as well as few clinical trials to support the efficacy of any treatment. The negative organoleptic perceptions associated with dysphagia diets further exacerbate undernutrition and malnutrition. Over the years, scientist in food science, nutritionists, psychologists and other health professionals have proposed parameters when formulating novel foods for the treatment of dysphagia. Beyond the nutritional composition of adapted foods for the treatment of dysphagia, this chapter will present multidimensional factors affecting food intake, sensory evaluations, rheological parameters as well as the available research to date with respect to optimizing nutritional treatment of dysphagia. To date, extrapolation to everyday food formulations remains a real challenge. To ensure success, thorough, individualized nutritional care plans need to be implemented and monitored regularly. An international knowledge transfer database must be considered to help document the innovations proposed in texture-modified foods and thickened fluids in order to benefit patients of all ages and origins.

Keywords: nutrition, rheology, sensory evaluation, dysphagia

1. Introduction

The contextual application and impact of nutritional interventions in the clinical treatment of dysphagia have been studied in the scientific literature [1–4]. Articles published as early as 1946 are presenting difficulties in swallowing due to either tonsillectomy, achalasia, myasthenia gravis, dysphagia lusoria—vascular compression of the esophagus—malignant causes and focused mainly on the esophageal phase of food ingestion [5–8]. An interest in difficulty in chewing and eating was also brought forward in the 1960s by the challenges of swallowing in neurological diseases or post-stroke patients [9–11]. Nearly 60 years later, the complexity of food ingestion in adults afflicted by deglutition disorders, more specifically dysfunctions of the oral and oropharyngeal regions, continues to be an important clinical challenge. The multifaceted aspects of food perception, mastication, preparation and propulsion of the bolus for an effective deglutition is still a major preoccupation for patients, families and caregivers.

IntechOpen

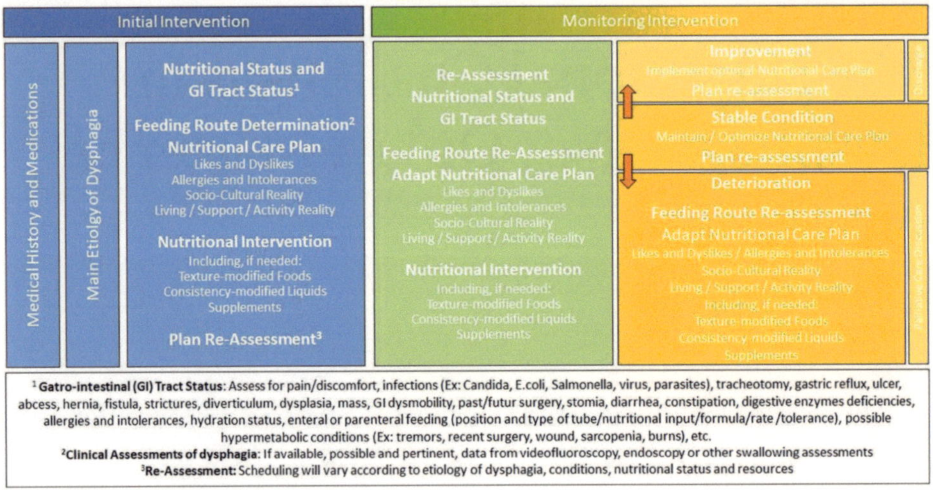

Figure 1.
Nutritional intervention route in dysphagia context.

The natural and reflex driven act of feeding one-self in adulthood is in fact an intricate emotional, sensory and neuromuscular achievement. It is directed by visual, olfactory, tactile and gustatory stimulations leading to pleasure and social interactions. Feeding one-self needs to meet much more than just pure physiological goals, particularly in healthcare.

> *"In spite of food fads, fitness programs, and health concerns, we must never lose sight of a beautifully conceived meal."*
>
> *– Julia Child.*

The difficulty to chew and swallow foods and liquids, known as dysphagia, often leads to malnutrition, impaired immune system and pneumonia [12–15]. In fact, presbyphagia (gradual and subtle decrease in swallowing capacity) and persistent undernutrition have been linked to sarcopenia and, more specifically pulmonary sarcopenia [16–20].

Several medical conditions such as head and neck cancers, cerebrovascular accidents, dementia, neurodegenerative diseases and aging could lead to dysphagia. Contingent to the underlying etiology and the evaluation/reporting method, reported prevalence of oropharyngeal dysphagia vary greatly, ranging from 11.4 to 91.7% in various assessed populations [21, 22]. Finally, dysphagia could improve, remain stable or worsen, needing recurrent assessments and adaptation of nutritional treatments (**Figure 1**). The conditions presenting some of the highest prevalence rates are observed in the very old frail populations presenting neurodegenerative conditions [21, 22].

2. Nutritional interventions

The past century has seen a remarkable evolution for human nutrition. Nutritional requirements for various population groups were adopted for different parts of the world and used to assess quality of food intake or food service delivery of well balanced meals in hospitals, schools, or daycare as well as or nutrition labeling of commercial food products [23–25]. Detailed nutritional values and composition of foods can now be more comprehensively assessed. Therefore, menus' macro and micronutrients are regularly being calculated for individual needs. Additionally, several databases exist to assess food intake in a wide array of clienteles (infants, children, athletes, elderly, etc.), food types or food service contexts [26–38].

It is regularly stated that, dysphagia leads to diminished food intake, poor functional status and increased risk of pneumonia. To improve the situation, foods and liquids are gradually adapted in texture or consistency to offer softer, moist and cohesive boluses and meet the needs of the patients' changing medical condition. In fact, it is now internationally recognized that various texture-modified foods (TMF) and thickened fluids (TF) are considered the cornerstone of clinical treatment and should be carefully evaluated [39]. Interestingly, in research studies investigation appetite and food intake in relationship to food oral processing, a meta-analysis published by Krop and colleagues noted that increased food oral processing (chewing) reduced food intake (−0.28 effect size; 95% CI: −0.36, 0.19; I2 statistic = 61.52%) and curbed appetite (−0.20 effect size; 95% CI: −0.30, 0.11; I2 statistic = 0%) [40]. Given this evidence, the decreased oral processing required to ingest TMF should be linked to improved oral food intake which is mostly sought after in dysphagia nutritional intervention. Additionally, thickening agents used to increase the consistency and reduce flow velocity are known to contribute to nutritional density [41]. So, shall we see an instant improvement? Not, according to the literature.

For the past 20 years, nutrient composition of institutional diets or TMF dysphagia diets have been repeatedly identified as deficient in energy and macro- or micronutrients [42–52] and remain a well known contributing factor of undernutrition and sarcopenia. Internationally, professional organizations are suggesting guidelines for better healthcare nutrition, including dysphagia nutritional care plans [53–57]. Fortification in energy, protein content or micronutrients of TMF, and the use of snacks are suggested to improve nutritional status [58–60]. But, sensory characteristics of TMF and TF such as taste, mouthfeel and appearance are regularly perceived negatively [61–65] and this nutritional treatment is seen as a psychosocial burden by staff and patients [66–71]. The challenge lies in adapting the foods offered to patients presenting dysphagia to optimize/improve nutritional content while maintain acceptable sensory characteristics!

Very few randomized clinical trials looking at comprehensive food intake reports for MTD and TF are found in the literature [72–74]. They were conducted in elderly populations, for a limited assessment time and are of small sample sizes. They did take in consideration complete dietary intakes, including oral nutritional supplements (ONS), meals and snacks. Detailed quantitative dietary assessments using weighed food records and done over several days in order to reflect usual intake are complex and time consuming [75]. This could explain the paucity of publications.

First in 2006, a small randomized controlled trial of 12 weeks was conducted by Germain et al. in frail elderly residents in a long-term care (LTC) facility (Treatment Group: n = 8; age: 82.5 ± 4.41 years, weight 55.9 ± 12.1 kg, BMI 22.4 ± 3.93; Control Group: n = 9; age, 84.6 ± 3.81 years, weight 54.3 ± 7.49 kg, BMI 21.2 ± 2.31). Prior to randomization, all participants were assessed for oropharyngeal of dysphagia and TMF and TF were prescribed as needed. The control group received usual TMF and the treatment group received reshaped pureed or minced foods. Intakes were calculated using 3-day weighed food records at Baseline, Midway and End points. The average weight in the treated group augmented compared to the control group (3.90 ± 2.30 vs. −0.79 ± 4.18 kg; $p = 0.02$). Furthermore, the treated group had an improved intake of total energy, proteins, fats, total saturated fats, monounsaturated fats, potassium, magnesium, calcium, phosphorus, zinc, vitamin B-2, and vitamin D compared to control subjects ($p \leq 0.05$) [72].

In 2017, following a 20-week intervention, Côté et al. also demonstrated improved intakes in a multi-center study of 15 elderly LTC residents (Treatment Group: n = 7). In this study, participants were assessed for oropharyngeal dysphagia to ensure adequate prescription level of TMF and TF. The control group received institutional TMF and the treatment group received reshaped pureed or minced foods (Épikura©). Proportions of food intakes were measured by comparing pictures of the content of the tray, before and after the meals (2 consecutive days; lunch and supper meals; excluding supplements and drinks). Although participants' body weights remained unchanged, the an increase in energy ($p = 0.004$), carbohydrate ($p = 0.04$) and lipid ($p = 0.001$) intakes in the treated group was documented [73].

Lastly in 2019, Reyes-Torres et al. implemented a controlled TMF and TF diet (n = 20 participants) to be compared to isocaloric standard diet (n = 20 participants) for 12 weeks. All participants received instructions in regards to swallowing rehabilitation techniques. Daily energy and protein intakes were assessed by 24-h multiple-step recalls and calculated using Food Processor Nutrition Analysis® software. In the intervention group, results revealed improved energy intakes (29 ± 10 to 40 ± 15 kcal/kg, $p = 0.009$) and protein intakes (1.3 ± 0.6 to 1.8 ± 0.7 g/kg, $p = 0.03$). Likewise, body weight were increased (56 ± 10 to 60 ± 10 kg, $p < 0.001$) as well as handgrip strength (18 ± 11 to 21 ± 13 kg, $p = 0.004$). Control group parameters remained unchanged. Therefore it appears that, although isocaloric to the standard pureed diet, better texture controlled pureed foods and TF allowed for improved dietary intakes and overall physical health status.

More recently, in a 12-week intervention study involving 50 elderly individuals living in a LTC facility (age: 89.12 ± 4.18 years), Rondanelli and colleagues also demonstrated that meal appreciation and nutritional status can be improved with tailored pureed texture meals [76]. This research team assessed meal intake with the Comstock Method of visual estimations of food waste [77] as an alternative to weighed dietary intake measures. It is noteworthy to mention that digital imaging methods to assess food intakes in various contexts (school cafeterias, restaurants, hospitals, etc.) have improved since their development in the early 1980s [78]. Visual estimations increasing used in research as they have the potential to help document food intake in larger groups with excellent agreement with the direct observational method, good agreement for between observers assessments comparison and presents very high intra-rater agreements [79–83].

Finally, in a case-crossover study published in 2022, Bayne et al. implemented sensory-enhanced, fortified snacks (quick-dissolving crisps, puree dips, and dry soup blends) for 8 weeks. The snacks improved the quality of nutritional intake among nursing home residents [84].

The presence and severity of dysphagia should prompt an individualized, nutritionally adequate and texture/consistency adapted nutritional interventions care plan to maintain or improve nutritional status and overall health of these patients. Although intuitively sound, few randomized clinical trials or interventions studies can be found using a clearly identified adapted nutritional intervention in association to specific severity of dysphagia. These rare and modest investigations seem to confirm that, other than using oral nutritional supplements, maintaining or improving nutritional density of foods provided by food services is possible. However, given the unfortunate poor quality of the research to date, systematic reviews repeatedly request more and better investigations [50, 54, 85, 86].

Admittedly, several confounding variables affect any nutritional research protocols: age groups, oropharyngeal or esophageal dysphagia, sample sizes, clinical settings, cultural reality, foods and ONS offered, number of meals assessed, dietary intake assessment method, duration of study, initial nutritional and clinical status, disparity in assessment approaches and measured outcomes, etc. The impact of nutritional interventions is challenging to measure (**Table 1**) [13, 76, 87–89]. Often, assessments have been conducted in elderly populations, possibly due to the convenience of studying cohorts in a more controlled environment. Conversely, clinical conclusions on the efficacy of these trials in younger populations should carefully extrapolated.

Sources	Participants	Assessment	Conclusion
Vucea et al. [13] (2018) Canada	Cross-sectional study Multi-center n = 337 Regular diet n = 139 Minced diet n = 68 Pureed diet Age = 86.8 ± 7.8 y 32 LTC facilities	MNA-SF InterRAI LTCF Cognitive Scale Ed-FED	MNA-SF score were lower for patients on MTF, dementia, ONS, assistance to fed or poor oral health MNA-SF score were higher for patients with micronutrient supplements or family assistance for meals. Malnutrition risk increased when diet texture prescription was changed from regular to minced diet Malnutrition risk increased when diet texture prescription was changed from regular to pureed diet
Shimizu et al. [87] (2020) Japan	Retrospective cohort Single-center n - 218 with pneumonia Age = 82.9 ± 9.8 y TMD group Multiple stages TMD (M-TMD) group	Food Intake Level Scale Japan TMD Scale MNA-SF	The M-TMD were related to the maintenance or improvement of swallowing capacity and nutritional status Note: *Nutritional intake not assessed* *Dysphagia severity not assessed*
Razalli et al. [88] (2021) Malaysia	Cross-sectional study Single-center n = 95 TMF diet Age: 64.2 ± 16.7 y Blended diet Mixed porridge diet Minced diet	1 day lunch (L) + dinner(D) Food waste Food appreciation Clinical/external factors such as appetite, assistance, time to eat, oral nutritional support	Blended diet Food waste—lunch: 68.8% Food waste—dinner: 63.3% Correlated with variety of food, time to eat meal and appetite Mixed porridge diet: Food waste—lunch: 36.3% Food waste—dinner: 33.9% Correlated with texture and temperature Minced diet: Food waste—lunch: 57.9% Food waste—dinner: 55.5% Correlated with appearance, taste, vegetables and chicken/meat/fish Note: *Nutritional intake not assessed* *Dysphagia severity not assessed*
Endo et al. [89] (2021) Japan	Longitudinal study Multi-center n = 284 Regular diet n = 171 TMF diet Age = 86.5 ± 7.8 y Duration = 1 year 25 LTC facilities	Severity of dysphagia Weight Barthelet Index Total energy intake Food form	ADL and change in food from regular to TMD form were associated to weight loss

Sources	Participants	Assessment	Conclusion
Rondanelli et al. [76] (2021) Italy	Intervention study Single-center n = 25 pureed diet 1223 kcal and 44 g protein per meal n = 25 consistency controlled MTD 1400 kcal and 53 g protein per meal All beverages are thickened Age = 89.2 ± 4.6 y	Meal satisfaction Food intake MNA Arm- and calf-circumferences Handgrip Blood chemistry *Dysphagia Outcome and Severity Scale (DOSS) as inclusion criteria*	Significant improvements were observed for food intake, meal appreciation, BMI, arm- and calf-circumferences, MNA, handgrip Prealbumin and albumin Folic acid, vitamin D and ionized calcium PCR and TNF-alpha Note: *Dysphagia severity was assessed but not used to stratify data*

Table 1.
Selected nutritional trials in adult patients presenting dysphagia.

Regrettably, dysphagia is too often considered as present or not present in research investigations. As an adapted nutritional individualized treatment, TMF and TF should be selected according to the level of severity of dysphagia. This variable is frequently ignored when evaluating the impact nutritional of treatments whether it is TMF, TF or ONS. Likewise, the severity level of the dysphagia is often extrapolated in observational or epidemiological studies by reporting descriptive aspects of TMF being served to patients [13, 90]. This premise could falsely assume that all participants had been properly assessed or monitored or that all foods were optimally controlled for their texture, consistency or nutrient density. Poorly assessing, documenting and reporting dysphagia severity scale in publications undoubtedly leads to inconsistent results and interpretation. An analogy with optometry assessments can be made. Optometrists will not report poor or good vision. Optometrists will report myopia or presbyopia in well-defined optical units called diopters. Individualized prescription will be proposed and corrective lenses will be provided. Although such precision in dysphagia severity assessment is still difficult to measure for all patients, it must be maintain as part of the assessment evaluation when conclusions are drawn from different trials.

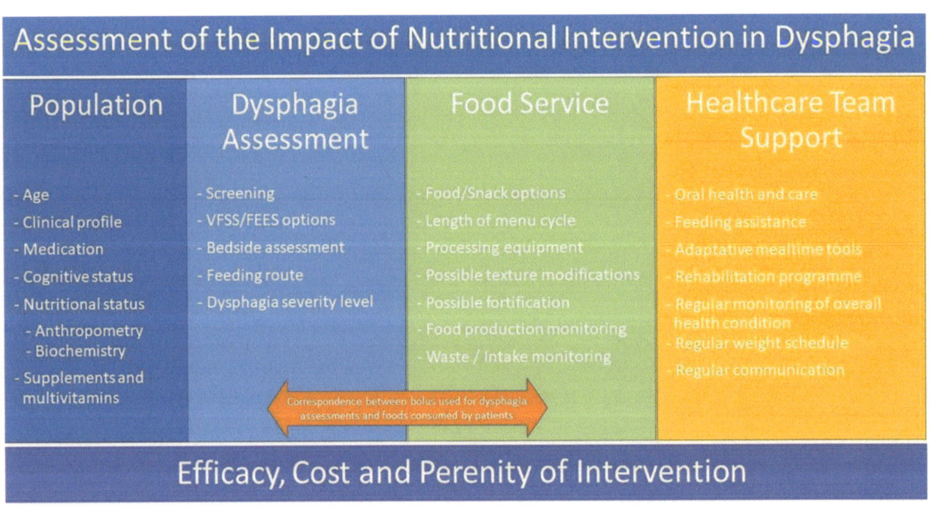

Figure 2.
Key factors for a meaningful nutritional intervention trial in dysphagia context.

Various dysphagia assessment tools exist: screening tools, bedside assessments or more sophisticated instrumental investigation methods such as surface electromyography (sEMG) biofeedback, manometry, videofluoroscopy or fiberoptic endoscopy evaluations. Clientele, clinical context or availability of expertise and equipment to conduct these tests will determine if they can used or not. Their usefulness and their validity continue to be challenged [91–97]. The

Dysphagia Outcome and Severity Scale [100] (1999) (United States)	DOSS	Design intended population: adult, post-stroke For videofluoroscopy or fiberendoscopy swallow study **Full per-oral nutrition (P.O): normal diet** Level 7: normal in all situations Normal diet No strategies or extra time needed Level 6: within functional limits/modified independence Normal diet, functional swallow Patient may have mild oral or pharyngeal delay, retention or trace epiglottal undercoating but independently and spontaneously compensates/clears May need extra time for meal Have no aspiration or penetration across consistencies **Full P.O.: modified diet and/or independence** Level 5: mild dysphagia: distant supervision, may need one diet consistency restricted May exhibit one or more of the following Aspiration of thin liquids only but with strong reflexive cough to clear completely Airway penetration midway to cords with one or more consistency or to cords with one consistency but clears spontaneously Retention in pharynx that is cleared spontaneously Mild oral dysphagia with reduced mastication and/or oral retention that is cleared spontaneously Level 4: mild–moderate dysphagia: Intermittent supervision/cueing, one or two consistencies restricted May exhibit one or more of the following Retention in pharynx cleared with cue Retention in the oral cavity that is cleared with cue Aspiration with one consistency, with weak or no reflexive cough Or airway penetration to the level of the vocal cords with cough with two consistencies Or airway penetration to the level of the vocal cords without cought with one consistency Level 3: moderate dysphagia: Total assist, supervision, or strategies, two or more diet consistencies restricted May exhibit one or more of the following Moderate retention in pharynx, cleared with cue Moderate retention in oral cavity, cleared with cue Airway penetration to the level of the vocal cords without cough with two or more consistencies Or aspiration with two consistencies, with weak or no reflexive cough Or aspiration with one consistency, no cough and airway penetration to cords with one, no cough **Non-oral nutrition necessary** Level 2: moderately severe dysphagia: Maximum assistance or use of strategies with partial P.O. only (tolerates at least one consistency safely with total use of strategies) May exhibit one or more of the following Severe retention in pharynx, unable to clear or needs multiple cues Severe oral stage bolus loss or retention, unable to clear or needs multiple cues Aspiration with two or more consistencies, no reflexive cough, weak volitional cough Or aspiration with one or more consistency, no cough and airway penetration to cords with one or more consistency, no cough Level 1: severe dysphagia: NPO: Unable to tolerate any P.O. safely May exhibit one or more of the following Severe retention in pharynx, unable to clear Severe oral stage bolus loss or retention, unable to clear Silent aspiration with two or more consistencies, nonfunctional volitional cough Or unable to achieve swallow

Functional Oral Intake Scale [101] (2005) (United States)	FOIS	Design intended population: adult, post-stroke **Tube dependent** Level 1: No oral intake Level 2: Tube dependent with minimal/inconsistent oral intake Level 3: Tube supplements with consistent oral intake **Total oral intake** Level 4: Total oral intake of a single consistency Level 5: Total oral intake of multiple consistencies requiring special preparation Level 6: Total oral intake with no special preparation, but must avoid specific foods or liquid items Level 7: Total oral intake with no restrictions
Eat Assessment Tool [102] (2008) (United States)	EAT-10	Design intended population: adult, various clinical diagnoses Developed by Expert Panel 10 questions pertaining to eating difficulty EAT-10 score of 3 or higher: abnormal
Food Intake LEVEL Scale [103] (2013) (Japan)	FILS	Design intended population: palliative care patients **No oral intake** Level 1: No swallowing training is performed except for oral care. Level 2: Swallowing training not using food is performed. Level 3: Swallowing training using a small quantity of food is performed. **Oral intake and alternative nutrition** Level 4: Easy-to-swallow food less than the quantity of a meal (enjoyment level) is ingested orally. Level 5: Easy-to-swallow food is orally ingested in one to two meals, but alternative nutrition is also given. Level 6: The patient is supported primarily by ingestion of easy-to-swallow food in three meals, but alternative nutrition is used as a complement. **Oral intake alone** Level 7: Easy-to-swallow food is orally ingested in three meals. No alternative nutrition is given. Level 8: The patient eats three meals by excluding food that is particularly difficult to swallow. Level 9: There is no dietary restriction, and the patient ingests three meals orally, but medical considerations are given. Level 10: There is no dietary restriction, and the patient ingests three meals orally (normal).

Table 2.
Scales of severity of dysphagia - assessment tools.

protocols for each evaluation differ. Bolus types and quantities consumed to perform the tests also differ. Additionally, diverse texture modifiers [65, 98] are used to change bolus consistency and texture of TMF and TF. In a clinical context, medications can also require consistency or texture modifications rendering new formulations which are also poorly understood [99]. Finally, and perhaps even more pertinent for nutritional interventions, no publication to date can be found providing a clear relationship between the various boluses provided during these assessments, the modification of consistency and texture occurring during the oropharyngeal phase of swallow and the multitude of foods possibly available at meals. Therefore, these investigation techniques must remain surrogate assessment methods of swallowing capacity and direct extrapolation of the capacity to prepare and swallow various types of bolus can only truly be monitored using a careful diagnostic process and impact of therapeutic approaches, in realistic contextual mealtime conditions, over time (**Figure 2**).

Keeping these limitations in mind, scales evaluating severity of oropharyngeal dysphagia have been validated with various clienteles. Examples of such scales would be the 7-point Dysphagia Outcome and Severity Scale (DOSS) [100], the 7-point Functional Oral Intake Scale (FOIS) [101], the Eating Assessment Tool (EAT-10) [102] and the 10-point observer-rating scale Food Intake LEVEL Scale (FILS) [103] (**Table 2**). Dysphagia severity scales are hardly ever applied in nutritional interventions or trials. But in 2006, Clavé et al. found a strong correlation between malnutrition and the dysphagia inventory score in 46 participants with brain damage, 46 participants with neurodegenerative diseases and eight healthy volunteers [104]. It could be helpful in future research focused on nutritional interventions to include a severity scale and determine if a correspondence is detectable between nutritional status and dysphagia severity.

Given all the existent caveats limiting the bedside and clinical assessment of dysphagia, nutritional interventions need to be prescribed to alleviate and compensate for the decrease in food intake. Notwithstanding the possible enteral nutritional avenue, texture modified diets, oral nutritional supplements, enriched snacks are some of the options proposed [21, 50, 60, 76, 85, 86, 101, 105–117].

3. Influential factors associated to eating

Eating is indispensable for subsistence. Therefore, it is a crucial component of the evolution of the human kind. As part of the essential evolutionary process, eating has taken various forms and adaptation has been linked to our survival.

Food choices and eating patterns are affected by several key elements such as biological influences (appetite, taste, hunger), psychological influences (mood or stress), socio-cultural determinants (family, peers, income, skills) and learnt behaviors [118, 119]. Côté et al. have depicted multiple factors to consider when providing adapted foods to the elderly. These factors remain intact, if not more important, once dysphagia becomes symptomatic (**Figure 3**) [120].

In the context of texture-modified foods and thickened fluids for the nutritional treatment of dysphagia, thc apprcciation of foods is often described as a burden [49, 66, 70, 71, 86, 121]. The reasons behind this present state of affairs are very complex and possibly imbedded in human survival programming itself.

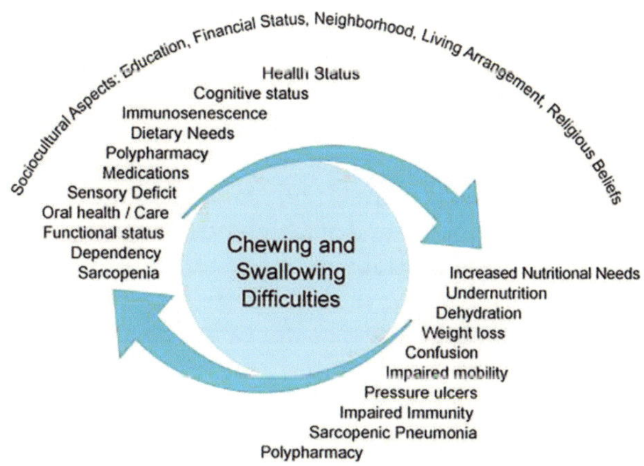

Figure 3.
Interaction model of key factors affecting feeding in the context of dysphagia in the older adult population.

4. Starting at the beginning: human evolution and food intake

The need of water and food was stated as a key necessity in the Maslow Hierarchy of Needs [122]. As humanoids evolved, the feeding techniques and the human chewing capabilities have evolved and adapted through time. Paleoanthropologist Dr. Rick Potts is the founder of the Human Origins Program at the Smithsonian's National Museum of Natural History, Washington, DC [123]. Potts describes the evolution of the human cranium developing from a small brain case and slope-like face to our current species with the largest brain case and the smallest face. The mandibular bone (not shown on the video) would have also changed in shape and strength affecting the capacity to chew foods and prepare the food bolus for swallowing.

Ledogar and colleagues [124] studied the morphology and the facial biomechanics of cranium specimens from various regions around the globe. Using computational biology, the research group created a model (named ALL-HUM) incorporating several characteristics of crania to which they allocated human bone tissue and masticatory muscle force values in order to predict cranial mechanics and calculate strains and bites forces of our ancestors. The masticatory gracilization over time of the human face was less stiff than the chimpanzee comparatives but were efficient in bite force application. These findings support the hypothesis that consumption of less mechanically challenging foods or the origination of extra-oral processing techniques (tools and cooking) accompanied these morphological changes. Humans adapted in several ways to evolved in various regions of the globe. One impressive adaptation was food preparation as well as feeding and chewing techniques as it is essential to survival of the species.

4.1 Taste perception

The biomechanics of human masticatory abilities are definitely important elements of feeding. However, feeding evolution is not only linked to our capacity to mechanically break down or process foods. It is associated to an array of sensations which also guide humans in accepting or refusing the ingestion of substances. It is believed that taste perception is an adaptive response [125] to assessing nutritional content or toxicity of foods. Initially believed to be spatially mapped on the tongue, it is now understood that taste receptors are found across the tongue [126]. In fact, located in the oropharyngeal region, the primary tastes of sweet, bitter, salty, sour and umami receptors could have helped humans in detecting acceptable foods sources. One type of taste receptor cell was identified for each of the sweet and umami tastes. For salt and sour tastes, possibly more than one are involved. However, bitter taste is detected by 25 different types of cell receptors [127, 128]. Therefore, primates and humans are capable to detect bitterness which prevents the consumption of possible toxic plants [129]. Animal studies have shown that, although specific taste buds regenerated at a high turnover rate, they maintain the capacity to reconnect to the central nervous system due to labeled line wiring. Essentially, labeled line wiring allows the bitter taste center to convey and perceive only bitter peripheral signal or the sweet center carry only sweet signal. The molecules responsible for directing these gustatory nerves are known as semaphorins and are proteins involved in neuronal axon guidance which permit high specificity [130–133]. Consequently in humans, taste perception is highly regulated and neurologically wired to allow innocuous ingestion of a wide array of substances.

New investigations pertaining to the microbiome have associated oral microbiota composition and with taste perception and reported food intake. Although providing exploratory results, it is proposed that the oral microbiota could also be affecting taste and smell perception as well as overall appetite [134–140].

4.2 Mouthfeel and texture perception

Ingestion of food is also guided by mouthfeel and texture perceptions as well as appreciation of the masticated bolus. Oral processing is a complex progression of neuromuscular interactions which prepares and assess food prior to swallowing. As food is being broken down and imbibed with saliva, it is in contact with the oral sensory receptors and an integrated sensory evaluation of tastes, volatile compounds and texture will occur [141, 142].

Electromyography (EMG) has been used to assess electric activity of the main masticatory muscles in healthy participants. Coupled to chewing cycle counts, tongue mobility, tongue pressure, salivation or videofluoroscopy studies, the mechanistic involved pre- and peri-swallowing can be assessed [143–148]. In a study looking at gels and sols, muscle activity required until swallowing appeared to be well correlated with the required force deployed for large compression deformation which occurs at the initiation of mastication [145]. Tournier and colleagues observed large inter-participant variation both for salivation and oral processing after 5 healthy participants masticated 4 breads of different textures and compositions [146]. Mori and colleagues studied the laterality of the posterior tongue movement in 20 young and health adults by [147]. Gummy jelly, sponge cake and mashed potatoes were assessed as representative of gradient mastication intensity requirements at the initiation, middle and end of mastication stages. For the purpose of the study, the participants were asked to masticate only on the right side or only on the left side. They measured a more intense EMG activity on the side of mastication for the gummy jelly and documented that tongue activity was affected by the food texture. Finally, Matsuo and colleagues investigated the masticatory function of 22 young participants an 32 community-dwelling older individuals of either normal or oral hypofunction. For their investigation, the test samples were a control meatloaf, meatloaf containing lotus root, control chicken ball or chicken ball with almonds slivers (10 g per bite). The documented mean EMG amplitudes and integrated EMG activity were lower for control samples which were softer test foods. Oral functions, including dental condition, appeared to decline with age and would have influenced the assessed mastication capacity [148].

The characterization of the biomechanics of bolus preparation and its impact on swallowing capacity is still being investigated [149–151] and remains limited in application for daily clinical investigations or association to diversified menu items around the globe. Few foods have been assessed. However, the variability in bolus process are highlighted and the impact could be important.

Individual physiognomy, quality of dentition and capacity to prepare foods for deglutition are only one part of the complex equation. The foods and liquids consumed bring their share of complexity. The lubrication of the bolus is also dependent on salivation. Intra-oral assessment of bolus texture and correlation to sensory perceptions are challenging.

5. Development of adapted texture-modified foods

5.1 Sensory evaluation

Acceptance by consumers of food products is a main priority for the food industry. Development of new products is time consuming and costly. However, the formal study of sensory evaluation of foods is a science with a relatively recent history. As stated by M.A. Drake, sensory evaluation is a "collection of techniques that seek to differentiate between a range of products based on all of their sensory

Like extremely
Like very much
Like moderately
Like slightly
Neither like nor dislike
Dislike slightly
Dislike moderately
Dislike very much
Dislike extremely

Table 3.
9-point hedonic scale [157].

characteristics and to determine a quantitative description of all the sensory attributes that can be identified, not just the defects" [152]. Methods such as discrimination testing (Is there a difference between 2 formulations?), acceptability (Which food would you prefer? Rating scales of relative dislike and like), descriptive sensory evaluation (How can we discriminate between a range of products based on all of their sensory characteristics?) have provided additional tools for application in research, product development, and marketing [152, 153]. Important developments in the science of sensory evaluation were initially triggered in the U.S. by the desire to optimize food intake in U.S. armed forces [152, 154–156]. With the creation of the food acceptance program in 1945, the U.S. Army Quartermaster Food and Container Institute (Chicago) had four main divisions which were food habit studies, psycho-physiological studies, organoleptic studies and statistical theory. In 1949 and 1950, psychologists David Peryam and Norman Girardot were hired to lead the Food Acceptance Research Branch. As measurement is essential to building comparative datasets, the staple nine-point hedonic scale (**Table 3**) was developed to assess food acceptance and preference [157, 158]. This scale remains in use today to asses customers appreciation of assorted food products such as chips [159], beef sausage using pigeon pea as binding agent [160] or yoghurt [161].

In the past, food development for the treatment of dysphagia customarily stemmed from clinical settings [44, 72, 162]. Researchers state that TMF and TF are deemed to be at the core of the nutritional treatment for dysphagia diets [65, 163], therefore, it is essential to evaluate the sensory profile if optimal ingestion is to be achieved. Limited publications have assessed sensory characteristics of TMF or TF. Pureed peaches [164], pureed carrots [165–167], meats [166, 167], soups, pates and timbales [167] were assessed primarily by healthy young adult for sensory perception. Thickened fluids have been studied more extensively: water with and without barium, lemon flavored water, juices, milk and infant formula [63, 168, 169]. But, even fewer publications have included participants with impaired swallowing [164, 166]. Studies are mainly conducted with the participation of young healthy adults. To be fair, several neurological diseases affect oral expression or comprehension of instructions which could render consumer assessments difficult. However, when recommending approaches to improve nutritional intakes and adherence to a proposed dysphagia diet, customer appreciation—likes and aversions of patients—should be at the core of the plan. More sensory research should be done with TMF and TF to help in developing complete, nutritious, appetizing and varied menu plans.

5.2 Rheological evaluation

Nutritional interventions for the treatment of dysphagia can take various forms and should progress with the medical conditions. Foods are molecularly and structurally elaborate and diverse. Oral nutritional supplements, texture-modified foods and thickened fluids often require the addition of the texture modifying agents which only adds to the complexity of these matrices. Comparing foods items is challenging in clinical trials. Over time, terminology and assessment methods have been proposed [170]. Two major milestones in the evolution of dysphagia diets development were the National Dysphagia Diet (NDD) [171] in 1999 and the International Dysphagia Diet Standardization Initiative (IDDSI) [39] in 2015.

Based on the work of food scientists Russell H. Mills [172] and Don Tymchuck [173], the NDD was the first diet to propose a quantifiable measure to assess flow of TF. Viscosity ranges were determine to discern different 3 different levels of consistency for fluids. Concepts of food texture such as adhesiveness, cohesiveness, firmness and springiness were also suggested to describe and classify TMF in 3 categories (**Table 4**).

After an extensive literature review and consultation among researchers, clinicians and industry leaders, the IDDSI group propose a more extensive descriptive framework and classification of the liquids with 5 levels to distinguish fluids and 5 levels for the MTF. A gravity flow test using a syringe is propose to measure liquid flow and 4 levels are recommended (**Table 4**). The syringe was preferred to other methods such as shear viscosity measurements or the use of empirical tests such as the Bostwick consistometer [174] or the line spread test due to the accessibility and ease of use of the syringe. But, velocity results obtained for various fluids using the IDDSI syringe and the Bostwick consistometer are unexpected and the discriminating capacity of the IDDSI levels remain to be demonstrated (**Figure 4**). The food texture descriptive parameters are still suggested to explain the MTF. However, other guidelines such as particle size, spoon-tilt test, drip test, fork pressure test and visual cues were added.

Both frameworks had important repercussions in the research and industrial arenas. By proposing a standardized terminology and food classification systems, these approaches helped researchers, clinicians, patients as well as the food industry to classify foods and allow better description of clinical protocols and comparison

NDD[1]—terminology		**IDDSI[2]—terminology**	
Fluids units		Drinks units (ml after 10 s)	
Thin Nectar-like Honey-like Spoon-thick	1–50 cP[3] 50–350 cP 351– 1750 cP ≥1750 cP	Thin—level—0 Slightly thick—level—1 Mildly thick—level—2 Moderately thick—level—3 Extremely thick—level—4	≤1 ml 1–4 ml 4–8 ml 8–10 ml ≥10 ml
Foods		Foods	
NDD level 1: dysphagia-pureed		Liquidized—level—3	8–10 ml
NDD level 2: dysphagia-mechanical altered		Pureed—level—4	≥10 ml
NDD level 3: dysphagia-advanced		Minced & moist—level—5	Transitional foods
Regular		Soft & bite-sized—level—6	
		Easy to chew-regular—level—7	

[1]*National dysphagia diet.*
[2]*International dysphagia diet standardization initiative.*
[3]*centiPoise.*

Table 4.
Terminology and rheological parameters associated to various levels of dysphagia diets.

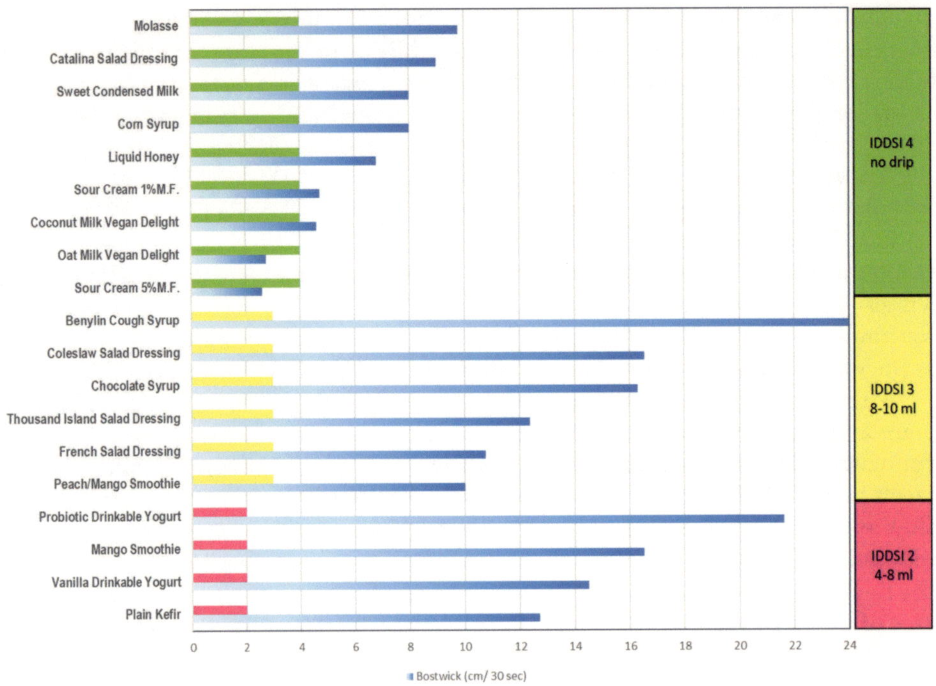

Figure 4.
Bostwick flow test and syringe flow test of common products (AAFC—Saint-Hyacinthe Research and Development Center (Canada)—unpublished data).

of interventions. Still, clinical trials will be required to assess their impact on nutritional status of patients suffering from dysphagia. The main novelty of these proposed frameworks was the use of rheology.

Rheology is the science of deformation and flow of matter [175]. In the context of oropharyngeal dysphagia, fluids and semi-solid foods are the object of interest. Two (2) extensive reviews helped the understanding of the science of rheology specifically in the perspective of oropharyngeal dysphagia treatment [176, 177].

First, the review published by Gallegos et al. [176] focused on the rheology of fluids. Providing a short review of basic rheological concepts, they present fundamental parameters impacting the flow of fluids such as stress, strain and strain rate (**Table 5**), type of fluids Newtonian, non-Newtonian, viscoplastic fluids as well as time-dependent viscous flow behavior, shear viscosity and extensional viscosity. In light of their work, it becomes evident that a bolus will undergo major pressure and deformation before and during the course of deglutition. The various forces applied (i.e. shear rates) throughout swallowing are challenging to measure and have not been clearly established. For the moment, a shear rate of 50 s^{-1} is generally used in the

Variable	Description	Units
Stress (τ or σ)	Force per unit area	Pascals (Pa)
Strain (ϒ)	Relative variation of position in the flow direction	Non dimensional
Strain rate (‘ϒ)	Strain variation over time	s^{-1}

These variables are temperature, pH, pressure and time dependent in Non-Newtonian fluids.
Swallowing imposes a stress on the bolus and deformation of the fluid occurs. The composition of the bolus will influenced its rheological behavior.

Table 5.
Fundamental dynamic and kinematic variables of flow [176].

literature. Salivary alpha-amylase and the presence of contrast fluids (barium) are also addressed since their presence impacts the bolus texture parameters and rheological behavior as the bolus is being processed orally prior or during swallowing.

Raheem and colleagues proposed a comprehensive review of the publications addressing the TMF. They present the various tests, both sensory and instrumental, available to the food industry to measure textural characteristics of foods. Similarly to the work done with TF, the rheological assessment of TMF is scare in the literature. According to this review, a better understanding of the complex food matrices used in the nutritional treatment of dysphagia, by all stakeholders, must take place to improve TMF.

5.3 Bridging the gaps

As early as 1963, Dr. Alina Szczesniak [178, 179] led the food industry in bridging the gap between the emerging technologies of the times and the sensory evaluations of foods. By developing standard rating scale to describe the mechanical characteristics of foods that were now assessed by texturemeters, Dr. Szczesniak demonstrated that although more repeatable and quantifiable, the data obtained for instruments remained insignificant in product development if they were not linked to human assessment and ratings. This vision of correlating instrumental and sensory assessments should inspire more future research in nutritional treatment for dysphagia. The recent 'mouthfeel wheel' terminology should be a step in the right direction [180].

6. Conclusion

Dysphagia is a condition affecting dietary intake. Although often underestimated, chronic undernutrition can exacerbate frailty and can lead to poor physical condition, declined immune system, sarcopenia and pneumonia. In view of the current literature, nutritional content, texture and consistency as well as appearance of texture-modified foods should be improved. An assortment of foods and fluids should be investigated to reflect more realistic food intake patterns. Above all, a personalized nutritional intervention is essential to prevent health decline.

Eating is indispensable to subsistence in addition to being a critical part of the social aspect of life. New texture-modified foods should be developed with the involvement of individuals affected by dysphagia to improve taste, textural profiles and overall acceptability. Clinical trials should improve documentation of the dysphagia severity level, nutritional intervention (foods/fluids offered) and food intake prescribed, nutrient density, satisfaction of meals and adaptation to patients nutritional needs. Research done to date, although essential to understanding this complex health issue, is still theoretical and lacks integration of expertise. We must improve clients/patients consultation. A large number of foods and fluids are required to build an nutritious and appealing menu which is an essential element to improve intakes. An open-sourced international clinical database for nutritional interventions in dysphagia, similar to existing food composition databases [181–184], would be a valuable tool to build a strong resource base. While archiving details of various food or fluids formulations, nutritional values and rheological parameters (when available), this compendium would support knowledge transfer and benefit food/pharmaceutical industries, researchers, clinicians as well as clients.

Finally, clinicians and research teams must continue to progress in bridging the knowledge gap between the foods used to evaluate dysphagia severity (with and without barium), the foods and the fluids available for nutritional interventions and recommendations for the development of commercial foods available for oropharyngeal dysphagia treatment.

Acknowledgements

First, I wish to thank Sophie Turcot for her support in organizing and maintaining our laboratory facilities as well as her reliability and diligence in her scientific work. I wish to acknowledge Francis Villeneuve for his methodical approach in the multiple rheological tests conducted. Finally, I wish to extend my most sincere gratitude to Amélie Giroux, Patricia Décarie and Vivianne Chagnon of the *Association professionnelle des nutritionnistes experts en dysphagie* for their patient-centered approach to clinical nutrition.

Conflict of interest

The authors declare no conflict of interest.

Notes/thanks/other declarations

The author is co-inventor of the CA2467625C patent. The current assignee of this patent is Her Majesty the Queen in Right of Canada.

Author details

Isabelle Germain
Saint-Hyacinthe Research and Development Centre, Agriculture and Agri-Food Canada, Saint-Hyacinthe, QC, Canada

*Address all correspondence to: isabelle.germain2@agr.gc.ca

References

[1] Ninfa A, Crispiatico V, Pizzorni N, Bassi M, Casazza G, Schindler A, et al. The care needs of persons with oropharyngeal dysphagia and their informal caregivers: A scoping review. PLoS ONE. 2021;**16**(9 September):1-20. DOI: 10.1371/journal.pone.0257683

[2] Rodd BG, Tas AA, Taylor KDA. Dysphagia, texture modification, the elderly and micronutrient deficiency: A review. Critical Reviews in Food Science and Nutrition. 2021:2-16. DOI: 10.1080/10408398.2021.1913571

[3] Ueshima J, Momosaki R, Shimizu A, Motokawa K, Sonoi M, Shirai Y, et al. Nutritional assessment in adult patients with dysphagia: A scoping review. Nutrients. 2021;**13**(3):1-15. DOI: 10.3390/nu13030778

[4] Wakabayashi H, Kishima M, Itoda M, Fujishima I, Kunieda K, Ohno T, et al. Diagnosis and treatment of sarcopenic dysphagia: A scoping review. Dysphagia. 2021;**36**(3):523-531. DOI: 10.1007/s00455-021-10266-8

[5] Gross RE. Surgical treatment for dysphagia lusoria. Annals of Surgery. 1946;**124**:532-534. DOI: 10.1097/00000658-194609000-00008

[6] Johnstone AS. Dysphagia due to causes other than malignant disease. Edinburgh Medical Journal. 1946;**53**:160-172

[7] Stinson WD. Myasthenia gravis of muscles of deglutition. Memphis Medical Journal. 1946;**21**:120

[8] Thorpe PA. A case of dysphagia in a woman of 78 cured by tonsillectomy. British Medical Journal. 1946;**1**(4453):723. DOI: 10.1136/bmj.1.4453.723

[9] Jones FA. Dysphagia. The Practitioner. 1946;**157**:219-221

[10] Kalinovskaya IY, Lavrova SV. Disorders of deglutition in some diseases of the central nervous system (Russian). Klinicheskaia Meditsina. 1973;**51**(9):69-74

[11] Jones RF. Stroke rehabilitation. Part II. Special considerations. The Medical Journal of Australia. 1975;**2**(21):799-801. DOI: 10.5694/j.1326-5377.1975.tb106314.x

[12] Eglseer D, Lohrmann C. Dysphagia and malnutrition in older hospitalized adults. Aktuel Ernahr Med. 2016;**41**(6):450-455. DOI: 10.1055/s-0042-119779

[13] Vucea V, Keller HH, Morrison JM, Duizer LM, Duncan AM, Carrier N, et al. Modified texture food use is associated with malnutrition in long term care: An analysis of making the Most of mealtimes (M3) project. The Journal of Nutrition, Health & Aging. 2018;**22**(8):916-922. DOI: 10.1007/s12603-018-1016-6

[14] Kiesswetter E, Hengeveld LM, Keijser BJ, Volkert D, Visser M. Oral health determinants of incident malnutrition in community-dwelling older adults. Journal of Dentistry. 2019;**85**:73-80. DOI: 10.1016/j.jdent.2019.05.017

[15] Furuya J, Suzuki H, Hidaka R, Nakagawa K, Yoshimi K, Nakane A, et al. Factors related to oral intake of food by hospitalized patients with malnutrition under the care of a nutrition support team. International Journal of Environmental Research and Public Health. 2021;**18**(21):1-11. DOI: 10.3390/ijerph182111725

[16] Hansen T, Nielsen RL, Houlind MB, Tavenier J, Rasmussen LJH, Jørgensen LM, et al. Dysphagia prevalence, time course, and association with probable sarcopenia, inactivity, malnutrition, and disease status in older patients admitted to an emergency

department: A secondary analysis of cohort study data. Geriatrics (Switzerland). 2021;**6**(2):1-14. DOI: 10.3390/GERIATRICS6020046

[17] Azzolino D, Damanti S, Bertagnoli L, Lucchi T, Cesari M. Sarcopenia and swallowing disorders in older people. Aging Clinical and Experimental Research. 2019;**31**(6):799-805. DOI: 10.1007/s40520-019-01128-3

[18] Wakabayashi H. Role of nutrition and rehabilitation in the prevention and management of sarcopenia and frailty. In: Recent Advances of Sarcopenia and Frailty in CKD. Singapore: Springer; 2020:117-138. DOI: 10.1007/978-981-15-2365-6_8

[19] Nagano A, Wakabayashi H, Maeda K, Kokura Y, Miyazaki S, Mori T, et al. Respiratory sarcopenia and sarcopenic respiratory disability: Concepts, diagnosis, and treatment. The Journal of Nutrition, Health & Aging. 2021;**25**(4):507-515. DOI: 10.1007/s12603-021-1587-5

[20] de Sire A, Ferrillo M, Lippi L, Agostini F, de Sire R, Ferrara PE, et al. Sarcopenic dysphagia, malnutrition, and oral frailty in elderly: A comprehensive review. Nutrients. 2022;**14**(5):1-23. DOI: 10.3390/nu14050982

[21] Gallegos C, Brito-de la Fuente E, Clavé P, Costa A, Assegehegn G. Nutritional aspects of dysphagia management. Advances in Food and Nutrition Research. 2017;**81**:271-318. DOI: 10.1016/bs.afnr.2016.11.008

[22] Xavier JS, Gois ACB, de Carvalho Palhano Travassos L, Pernambuco L. Oropharyngeal dysphagia frequency in older adults living in nursing homes: An integrative review. CODAS. 2021;**33**(3):1-12. DOI: 10.1590/2317-1782/20202020153

[23] Tsuboyama-Kasaoka N, Takizawa A, Tsubota-Utsugi M, Nakade M, Imai E, Kondo A, et al. Dietary intake of nutrients with adequate intake values in the dietary reference intakes for Japanese. Journal of Nutritional Science and Vitaminology. 2013;**59**(6):584-595. DOI: 10.3177/jnsv.59.584

[24] Price MY, Preedy VR. Chapter 44 - Dietary Reference Values. In: Metabolism and Pathophysiology of Bariatric Surgery: Nutrition, Procedures, Outcomes and Adverse Effects. London: Elsevier Inc.; 2017. pp. 399-417. DOI: 10.1016/B978-0-12-804011-9.00030-3

[25] Powers HJ. Approaches to setting dietary reference values for micronutrients, and translation into recommendations. The Proceedings of the Nutrition Society. 2021;**80**(3):365-372. DOI: 10.1017/S0029665121000562

[26] Martin CL, Clemens J, Moshfegh AJ. Items designated as fortified: Food and nutrient database for dietary studies (FNDDS), 2015-2016. Journal of Food Composition and Analysis. 2019;**84**:1-4. DOI: 10.1016/j.jfca.2019.103255

[27] Delgado JA, Vandenberg B, Neer D, D'Adamo R. Emerging nutrient management databases and networks of networks will have broad applicability in future machine learning and artificial intelligence applications in soil and water conservation. Journal of Soil and Water Conservation. 2019;**74**(6):113A-118A. DOI: 10.2489/JSWC.74.6.113A

[28] Van Puyvelde H, Perez-Cornago A, Casagrande C, Nicolas G, Versele V, Skeie G, et al. Comparing calculated nutrient intakes using different food composition databases: Results from the European prospective investigation into cancer and nutrition (EPIC) cohort. Nutrients. 2020;**12**(10):1-14. DOI: 10.3390/nu12102906

[29] Pompeu J, Gerage J, Ometto J. A spatiotemporal database on the energy, macro and micro-nutrients from the

Brazilian agricultural production. Data in Brief. 2020;**30**:1-13. DOI: 10.1016/j.dib.2020.105602

[30] Pehrsson PR, Mitchell DC. Advancing food and nutrient databases through partnerships and technology. Journal of Food Composition and Analysis. 2020;**92**:1-2. DOI: 10.1016/j.jfca.2020.103527

[31] Jasthi B, Pettit J, Harnack L. Addition of gluten values to a food and nutrient database. Journal of Food Composition and Analysis. 2020;**85**:1-4. DOI: 10.1016/j.jfca.2019.103330

[32] Fairulnizal M, Gunasegavan RDN, Khalid NM, Balasubramaniam V, Mustar S, Rashed AA. Recent techniques in nutrient analysis for food composition database. Molecules. 2020;**25**(19):1-45. DOI: 10.3390/molecules25194567

[33] Ma P, Li A, Yu N, Li Y, Bahadur R, Wang Q , et al. Application of machine learning for estimating label nutrients using USDA Global Branded Food Products Database, (BFPD). Journal of Food Composition and Analysis. 2021;**100**:1-9. DOI: 10.1016/j.jfca.2021.103857

[34] Rodrigues MP, Khandpur N, Fung TT, Sampson L, Oliveira MRM, Willett WC, et al. Development of DietSys: A comprehensive food and nutrient database for dietary surveys. Journal of Food Composition and Analysis. 2021;**102**:1-8. DOI: 10.1016/j.jfca.2021.104030

[35] Miller V, Singh GM, Onopa J, Reedy J, Shi P, Zhang J, et al. Global Dietary Database 2017: Data availability and gaps on 54 major foods, beverages and nutrients among 5.6 million children and adults from 1220 surveys worldwide. BMJ Global Health. 2021;**6**(2):1-19. DOI: 10.1136/bmjgh-2020-003585

[36] Drewnowski A. Plant-based milk alternatives in the USDA branded food products database would benefit from nutrient density standards. Nature Food. 2021;**2**(8):567-569. DOI: 10.1038/s43016-021-00334-5

[37] Ložnjak Švarc P, Jensen MB, Langwagen M, Poulsen A, Trolle E, Jakobsen J. Nutrient content in plant-based protein products intended for food composition databases. Journal of Food Composition and Analysis. 2022;**106**:1-10. DOI: 10.1016/j.jfca.2021.104332

[38] Pickford C, McCormack L, Liu Y, Eicher-Miller HA. US Department of agriculture food composition databases, the food and nutrient database for dietary studies 2013-2014, and the national nutrient database for standard reference version 28 yield significantly different nutrient totals of food items from eight midwestern food pantry inventories. Journal of the Academy of Nutrition and Dietetics. 2022 (In Press, Corrected Proof):1-10. DOI: 10.1016/j.jand.2022.01.010

[39] Martineau C. International dysphagia diet standardisation initiative: IDDSI framework. Médecine des Maladies Métaboliques. 2015;**13**(1):101-102. DOI: 10.1016/S1957-2557(19)30036-7

[40] Krop EM, Hetherington MM, Nekitsing C, Miquel S, Postelnicu L, Sarkar A. Influence of oral processing on appetite and food intake—A systematic review and meta-analysis. Appetite. 2018;**125**:253-269. DOI: 10.1016/j.appet.2018.01.018

[41] Miranda D, Breda J, Cardoso R, Gonçalves N, Caldas AC, Ferreira JJ. Should the energy contribution of commercial thickeners be considered in the nutrition plan of patients with dysphagia? Nutrition in Clinical Practice. 2020;**35**(4):649-654. DOI: 10.1002/ncp.10408

[42] Wright L, Cotter D, Hickson M, Frost G. Comparison of energy and

protein intakes of older people consuming a texture modified diet with a normal hospital diet. Journal of Human Nutrition and Dietetics. 2005;**18**(3):213-219. DOI: 10.1111/j.1365-277X.2005.00605.x

[43] Patricia Viganó C, Nilian Silva S, Camila Cremonezi J, Guilherme Vannucchi P, Marta CM. Variation in the energy and macronutrient contents of texture modified hospital diets. Revista Chilena de Nutricion. 2011;**38**(4): 451-457. DOI: 10.4067/S0717-75182011000400008

[44] Rocamora JAI, García-Luna PP. Texture modified diet; digestibility, nutritional value, and contributions to menu of hospitals and nursing homes. Nutrición Hospitalaria. 2014;**29**(4):873-879. DOI: 10.3305/nh.2014.29.4.7285

[45] Ettinger L, Keller HH, Duizer LM. Characterizing commercial pureed foods: Sensory, nutritional, and textural analysis. Journal of Nutrition in Gerontology and Geriatrics. 2014;**33**(3):179-197. DOI: 10.1080/21551197.2014.927304

[46] Ilhamto N, Keller HH, Duizer LM. The effect of varying ingredient composition on the sensory and nutritional properties of a pureed meat and vegetable. Journal of Nutrition in Gerontology and Geriatrics. 2014;**33**(3):229-248. DOI: 10.1080/21551197.2014.927307

[47] Keller HH, Carrier N, Slaughter SE, Lengyel C, Steele CM, Duizer L, et al. Prevalence and determinants of poor food intake of residents living in long-term care. Journal of the American Medical Directors Association. 2017;**18**(11):941-947. DOI: 10.1016/j.jamda.2017.05.003

[48] Keller HH, Lengyel C, Carrier N, Slaughter SE, Morrison J, Duncan AM, et al. Prevalence of inadequate micronutrient intakes of Canadian long-term care residents. The British Journal of Nutrition. 2018;**119**(9):1047-1056. DOI: 10.1017/S0007114518000107

[49] Maeda K, Ishida Y, Nonogaki T, Shimizu A, Yamanaka Y, Matsuyama R, et al. Burden of premorbid consumption of texture modified diets in daily life on nutritional status and outcomes of hospitalization. The Journal of Nutrition, Health & Aging. 2019;**23**(10):973-978. DOI: 10.1007/s12603-019-1237-3

[50] Wu XS, Miles A, Braakhuis A. Nutritional intake and meal composition of patients consuming texture modified diets and thickened fluids: A systematic review and metaanalysis. Healthcare (Basel). 2020;**8**(4):1-24. DOI: 10.3390/healthcare8040579

[51] Wu S, Morrison-Koechl J, Lengyel C, Carrier N, Awwad S, Keller H. Are therapeutic diets in long-term care affecting resident food intake and meeting their nutritional goals? Canadian Journal of Dietetic Practice and Research. 2020;**81**(4): 186-192. DOI: 10.3148/cjdpr-2020-015

[52] Sorensen J, Fletcher H, Macdonald B, Whittington-Carter L, Nasser R, Gramlich L. Canadian hospital food service practices to prevent malnutrition. Canadian Journal of Dietetic Practice and Research. 2021;**82**(4):167-175. DOI: 10.3148/cjdpr-2021-013

[53] Strowd L, Kyzima J, Pillsbury D, Valley T, Rubin B. Dysphagia dietary guidelines and the rheology of nutritional feeds and barium test feeds. Dysphagia. 2009;**24**(1):119-120. DOI: 10.1007/s00455-008-9191-y

[54] Beck AM, Kjaersgaard A, Hansen T, Poulsen I. Systematic review and evidence based recommendations on texture modified foods and thickened liquids for adults (above 17 years) with oropharyngeal dysphagia—An updated

clinical guideline. Clinical Nutrition. 2018;**37**(6):1980-1991. DOI: 10.1016/j.clnu.2017.09.002

[55] Thibault R, Abbasoglu O, Ioannou E, Meija L, Ottens-Oussoren K, Pichard C, et al. ESPEN guideline on hospital nutrition. Clinical Nutrition. 2021;**40**(12):5684-5709. DOI: 10.1016/j.clnu.2021.09.039

[56] Dziewas R, Michou E, Trapl-Grundschober M, Lal A, Arsava EM, Bath PM, et al. European Stroke Organisation and European Society for Swallowing Disorders guideline for the diagnosis and treatment of post-stroke dysphagia. European Stroke Journal. 2021;**6**(3):LXXXIX-CXV. DOI: 10.1177/23969873211039721

[57] Volkert D, Beck AM, Cederholm T, Cruz-Jentoft A, Hooper L, Kiesswetter E, et al. ESPEN practical guideline: Clinical nutrition and hydration in geriatrics. Clinical Nutrition. 2022;**41**(4):958-989. DOI: 10.1016/j.clnu.2022.01.024

[58] Kennewell S, Kokkinakos M. Thick, cheap and easy: Fortifying texture-modified meals with infant cereal. Nutrition and Dietetics. 2007;**64**(2): 112-115. DOI: 10.1111/j.1747-0080.2007.00101.x

[59] Ott A, Senger M, Lötzbeyer T, Gefeller O, Sieber CC, Volkert D. Effects of a texture-modified, enriched, and reshaped diet on dietary intake and body weight of nursing home residents with chewing and/or swallowing problems: An enable study. Journal of Nutrition in Gerontology and Geriatrics. 2019;**38**(4):361-376. DOI: 10.1080/21551197.2019.1628158

[60] Seemer J, Kiesswetter E, Fleckenstein-Sußmann D, Gloning M, Bader-Mittermaier S, Sieber CC, et al. Effects of an individualised nutritional intervention to tackle malnutrition in nursing homes: A pre-post study. European Geriatric Medicine. 2022;**13**:741-752. DOI: 10.1007/s41999-021-00597-y

[61] Matta Z, Chambers Iv E, Garcia JM, Helverson JM. Sensory characteristics of beverages prepared with commercial thickeners used for dysphagia diets. Journal of the American Dietetic Association. 2006;**106**(7):1049-1054. DOI: 10.1016/j.jada.2006.04.022

[62] Goldberg LR, Heiss CJ. The effect of appearance on the palatability of thickened apple juice: A pilot study. Topics in Clinical Nutrition. 2013;**28**(2):154-162. DOI: 10.1097/TIN.0b013e31828d79df

[63] Ong JJX, Steele CM, Duizer LM. Sensory characteristics of liquids thickened with commercial thickeners to levels specified in the International Dysphagia Diet Standardization Initiative (IDDSI) framework. Food Hydrocolloids. 2018;**79**:208-217. DOI: 10.1016/j.foodhyd.2017.12.035

[64] Munialo CD, Kontogiorgos V, Euston SR, Nyambayo I. Rheological, tribological and sensory attributes of texture-modified foods for dysphagia patients and the elderly: A review. International Journal of Food Science and Technology. 2020;**55**(5):1862-1871. DOI: 10.1111/ijfs.14483

[65] Schmidt HDOS, Komeroski MR, Steemburgo T, de Oliveira VR. Influence of thickening agents on rheological properties and sensory attributes of dysphagic diet. Journal of Texture Studies. 2021;**52**:587-602. DOI: 10.1111/jtxs.12596

[66] Ekberg O, Hamdy S, Woisard V, Wuttge-Hannig A, Ortega P. Social and psychological burden of dysphagia: Its impact on diagnosis and treatment. Dysphagia. 2002;**17**(2):139-146. DOI: 10.1007/s00455-001-0113-5

[67] Ilhamto N, Anciado K, Keller HH, Duizer LM. In-house pureed food

production in long-term care: Perspectives of dietary staff and implications for improvement. Journal of Nutrition in Gerontology and Geriatrics. 2014;**33**(3):210-228. DOI: 10.1080/21551197.2014.927306

[68] Austbø Holteng LB, Frøiland CT, Corbett A, Testad I. Care staff perspective on use of texture modified food in care home residents with dysphagia and dementia. Annals of Palliative Medicine. 2017;**6**(4):310-318. DOI: 10.21037/apm.2017.06.24

[69] Garcia JM, Chambers E, Russell EG, Katt A. Modifying food textures: Practices and beliefs of staff involved in nutrition care. American Journal of Speech-Language Pathology. 2018;**27**(4):1458-1473. DOI: 10.1044/2018_AJSLP-18-0021

[70] McCurtin A, Healy C, Kelly L, Murphy F, Ryan J, Walsh J. Plugging the patient evidence gap: What patients with swallowing disorders post-stroke say about thickened liquids. International Journal of Language & Communication Disorders. 2018;**53**(1):30-39. DOI: 10.1111/1460-6984.12324

[71] Steele SJ, Ennis SL, Dobler CC. Treatment burden associated with the intake of thickened fluids. Breathe. 2021;**17**(1):1-6. DOI: 10.1183/20734735.0003-2021

[72] Germain I, Dufresne T, Gray-Donald K. A novel dysphagia diet improves the nutrient intake of institutionalized elders. Journal of the American Dietetic Association. 2006;**106**(10):1614-1623. DOI: 10.1016/j.jada.2006.07.008

[73] Côté C, Payette H, Gagnon C. Prévenir la dénutrition des personnes âgées dysphagiques institutionnalisées avec une alimentation à textures adaptées: essai clinique randomisé. Canadian Journal of Dietetic Practice and Research. 2017;**78**(1):45-49. DOI: 10.3148/cjdpr-2016-031

[74] Reyes-Torres CA, Castillo-Martínez L, Reyes-Guerrero R, Ramos-Vázquez AG, Zavala-Solares M, Cassis-Nosthas L, et al. Design and implementation of modified-texture diet in older adults with oropharyngeal dysphagia: A randomized controlled trial. European Journal of Clinical Nutrition. 2019;**73**(7):989-996. DOI: 10.1038/s41430-019-0389-x

[75] Schoeller DA, Westerterp-Plantenga MS. Advances in the Assessment of Dietary Intake. United States: CRC Press; 2017. DOI: 10.1201/9781315152288

[76] Rondanelli M, Faliva MA, Peroni G, Perna S, Gasparri C, Fazia T, et al. A favorable effect on nutritional status of 12-week tailored texture-modified sous-vide cooking meals in institutionalized elderly women with oropharyngeal dysphagia: An intervention study. Minerva Endocrinology. 2021;**46**(2):202-213. DOI: 10.23736/S2724-6507.20.03232-0

[77] Comstock EM, St Pierre RG, Mackiernan YD. Measuring individual plate waste in school lunches. Visual estimation and children's ratings vs. actual weighing of plate waste. Journal of the American Dietetic Association. 1981;**79**(3):290-296

[78] Hawkins KR, Apolzan JW, Myers CA, Martin CK. The assessment of food intake with digital photography. In: Advances in the Assessment of Dietary Intake. United States: CRC Press; 2017. pp. 85-112. DOI: 10.1201/9781315152288

[79] Williamson DA, Allen HR, Martin PD, Alfonso AJ, Gerald B, Hunt A. Comparison of digital photography to weighed and visual estimation of portion sizes. Journal of the American Dietetic Association. 2003;**103**(9):1139-1145. DOI: 10.1016/S0002-8223(03)00974-X

[80] Martin CK, Han H, Coulon SM, Allen HR, Champagne CM, Anton SD. A novel method to remotely measure food intake of free-living individuals in real time: The remote food photography method. The British Journal of Nutrition. 2009;**101**(3):446-456. DOI: 10.1017/S0007114508027438

[81] Keller HH, Chambers LW, Fergusson DA, Niezgoda H, Parent M, Caissie D, et al. A mix of bulk and ready-to-use modified-texture food: Impact on older adults requiring dysphagic food. Canadian Journal on Aging. 2012;**31**(3):335-348. DOI: 10.1017/S0714980812000268

[82] Kawasaki Y, Kojima Y, Akamatsu R. Measuring patient dietary intake using visual estimation methods in Japanese hospitals: A qualitative study. Topics in Clinical Nutrition. 2016;**31**(4):335-345. DOI: 10.1097/TIN.0000000000000084

[83] Kawasaki Y, Kojima Y, Akamatsu R. Barriers to accurately measuring patients' dietary intake in hospitals using the visual estimation method: A qualitative study. International Journal of Health Care Quality Assurance. 2016;**29**(8):835-845. DOI: 10.1108/IJHCQA-04-2016-0042

[84] Bayne D, Barewal R, Shune SE. Sensory-enhanced, fortified snacks for improved nutritional intake among nursing home residents. Journal of Nutrition in Gerontology and Geriatrics. 2022;**41**(1):92-101. DOI: 10.1080/21551197.2022.2025971

[85] Essat M, Archer R, Williams I, Zarotti N, Coates E, Clowes M, et al. Interventions to promote oral nutritional behaviours in people living with neurodegenerative disorders of the motor system: A systematic review. Clinical Nutrition. 2020;**39**(8):2547-2556. DOI: 10.1016/j.clnu.2019.11.015

[86] Wu XS, Miles A, Braakhuis AJ. Texture-modified diets, nutritional status and mealtime satisfaction: A systematic review. Healthcare (Basel). 2021;**9**(6):1-19. DOI: 10.3390/healthcare9060624

[87] Shimizu A, Momosaki R, Kayashita J, Fujishima I. Impact of multiple texture-modified diets on Oral intake and nutritional status in older patients with pneumonia: A retrospective cohort study. Dysphagia. 2020;**35**(4):574-582. DOI: 10.1007/s00455-019-10063-4

[88] Razalli NH, Cheah CF, Mohammad NMA, Manaf ZA. Plate waste study among hospitalised patients receiving texture-modified diet. Nutrition Research and Practice. 2021;**15**(5):655-671. DOI: 10.4162/nrp.2021.15.5.655

[89] Endo A, Watanabe Y, Matsushita T, Okada K, Ohara Y, Iwasaki M, et al. Association between weight loss and food form in older individuals residing in long-term care facilities: 1-year multicenter longitudinal study. International Journal of Environmental Research and Public Health. 2021;**18**(20):1-10. DOI: 10.3390/ijerph182010776

[90] Namasivayam-Macdonald AM, Steele CM, Carrier N, Lengyel C, Keller HH. The relationship between texture-modified diets, mealtime duration, and dysphagia risk in long-term care. Canadian Journal of Dietetic Practice and Research. 2019;**80**(3):122-126. DOI: 10.3148/cjdpr-2019-004

[91] Steele CM, Molfenter SM, Bailey GL, Polacco RC, Waito AA, Zoratto DCBH, et al. Exploration of the utility of a brief swallow screening protocol with comparison to concurrent videofluoroscopy. Canadian Journal of Speech-Language Pathology & Audiology. 2011;**35**(3):228-242. DOI: 10.1007/s00455-010-9312-2

[92] Swan K, Cordier R, Brown T, Speyer R. Psychometric properties of

visuoperceptual measures of videofluoroscopic and fibre-endoscopic evaluations of swallowing: A systematic review. Dysphagia. 2019;**34**(1):2-33. DOI: 10.1007/s00455-018-9918-3

[93] Swan K, Cordier R, Brown T, Speyer R. Visuoperceptual analysis of the videofluoroscopic study of swallowing: An international Delphi study. Dysphagia. 2021;**36**(4):595-613. DOI: 10.1007/s00455-020-10174-3

[94] Edwards A, Froude E, Sharpe G, Carding P. Training for videofluoroscopic swallowing analysis: A systematic review. International Journal of Speech-Language Pathology. 2021;**23**(5):529-539. DOI: 10.1080/17549507.2020.1861327

[95] Speyer R, Cordier R, Sutt AL, Remijn L, Heijnen BJ, Balaguer M, et al. Behavioural interventions in people with oropharyngeal dysphagia: A systematic review and meta-analysis of randomised clinical trials. Journal of Clinical Medicine. 2022;**11**(3):1-31. DOI: 10.3390/jcm11030685

[96] Speyer R, Cordier R, Farneti D, Nascimento W, Pilz W, Verin E, et al. White paper by the European Society for Swallowing Disorders: Screening and non-instrumental assessment for dysphagia in adults. Dysphagia. 2022;**37**(2):333-349. DOI: 10.1007/s00455-021-10283-7

[97] Audag N, Goubau C, Toussaint M, Reychler G. Screening and evaluation tools of dysphagia in adults with neuromuscular diseases: A systematic review. Therapeutic Advances in Chronic Disease. 2019;**10**:1-15. DOI: 10.1177/2040622318821622

[98] Himashree P, Sengar AS, Sunil CK. Food thickening agents: Sources, chemistry, properties and applications—A review. International Journal of Gastronomy and Food Science. 2022;**27**:1-13. DOI: 10.1016/j.ijgfs.2022.100468

[99] Bravo-José P, Sáez-Lleó C, Moreno-Guillamont E. Combining liquid oral drugs with thickener: Compatibility and changes in viscosity. Dysphagia. 2021. Epub ahead of print. DOI: 10.1007/s00455-021-10348-7

[100] O'Neil KH, Purdy M, Falk J, Gallo L. The dysphagia outcome and severity scale. Dysphagia. 1999;**14**(3):139-145. DOI: 10.1007/PL00009595

[101] Crary MA, Carnaby Mann GD, Groher ME. Initial psychometric assessment of a functional oral intake scale for dysphagia in stroke patients. Archives of Physical Medicine and Rehabilitation. 2005;**86**(8):1516-1520. DOI: 10.1016/j.apmr.2004.11.049

[102] Belafsky PC, Mouadeb DA, Rees CJ, Pryor JC, Postma GN, Allen J, et al. Validity and reliability of the eating assessment tool (EAT-10). The Annals of Otology, Rhinology, and Laryngology. 2008;**117**(12):919-924. DOI: 10.1177/000348940811701210

[103] Kunieda K, Ohno T, Fujishima I, Hojo K, Morita T. Reliability and validity of a tool to measure the severity of dysphagia: The food intake LEVEL scale. Journal of Pain and Symptom Management. 2013;**46**(2):201-206. DOI: 10.1016/j.jpainsymman.2012.07.020

[104] Clavé P, De Kraa M, Arreola V, Girvent M, Farré R, Palomera E, et al. The effect of bolus viscosity on swallowing function in neurogenic dysphagia. Alimentary Pharmacology & Therapeutics. 2006;**24**(9):1385-1394. DOI: 10.1111/j.1365-2036.2006.03118.x

[105] Ninfa A, Pizzorni N, Eplite A, Moltisanti C, Schindler A. Validation of the Italian version of the functional oral intake scale (FOIS-It) against Fiberoptic endoscopic evaluation of swallowing and nutritional status. Dysphagia. 2022;**37**(1):137-147. DOI: 10.1007/s00455-021-10257-9

[106] Mortensen J, Pedersen AR, Nielsen JF, Kothari M. Construct and content validity of the functional oral intake scale; analyses from a cohort of patients with acquired brain injury. Brain Injury. 2020;**34**(9):1257-1263. DOI: 10.1080/02699052.2020.1800094

[107] Chen HJ, Chen JL, Chen CY, Lee M, Chang WH, Huang TT. Effect of an oral health programme on oral health, oral intake, and nutrition in patients with stroke and dysphagia in Taiwan: A randomised controlled trial. International Journal of Environmental Research and Public Health. 2019;**16**(12):1-12. DOI: 10.3390/ijerph16122228

[108] Hey C, Lange BP, Eberle S, Zaretsky Y, Sader R, Stover T, et al. Water swallow screening test for patients after surgery for head and neck cancer: Early identification of dysphagia, aspiration and limitations of oral intake. Dysphagia. 2014;**29**(3):405-406. DOI: 10.1007/s00455-014-9536-7

[109] Pinto AR, Cola PC, de Carvalho LR, Motonaga SM, da Silva RG. Oral intake and severity scale in neurogenic oropharyngeal dysphagia. Reviews in the Neurosciences. 2013;**21**(4):531-536. DOI: 10.4181/RNC.2013.21.798.6p

[110] Vucea V, Keller HH, Morrison JM, Duizer LM, Duncan AM, Steele CM. Prevalence and characteristics associated with modified texture food use in long term care: An analysis of making the most of mealtimes (M3) project. Canadian Journal of Dietetic Practice and Research. 2019;**80**(3):104-110. DOI: 10.3148/cjdpr-2018-045

[111] Seemer J, Kiesswetter E, Blawert A, Fleckenstein D, Gloning M, Bader-Mittermaier S, et al. An individualised nutritional intervention concept for nursing home residents with or at risk of malnutrition: An enable study. Geriatrics (Switzerland). 2021;**6**(1):1-12. DOI: 10.3390/geriatrics6010002

[112] Melgaard D, Westergren A, Skrubbeltrang C, Smithard D. Interventions for nursing home residents with dysphagia—A scoping review. Geriatrics (Switzerland). 2021;**6**(2):1-16. DOI: 10.3390/geriatrics6020055

[113] Bruno C, Collier A, Holyday M, Lambert K. Interventions to improve hydration in older adults: A systematic review and meta-analysis. Nutrients. 2021;**13**(10):1-20. DOI: 10.3390/nu13103640

[114] Huppertz VAL, van Wijk N, Baijens LWJ, de Groot LCPGM, Halfens RJG, Schols JMGA, et al. Design of the DYNAMO study: A multi-center randomized controlled trial to investigate the effect of pre-thickened oral nutritional supplements in nursing home residents with dysphagia and malnutrition (risk). BMC Geriatrics. 2020;**20**(1):1-10. DOI: 10.1186/s12877-020-01947-4

[115] Faccio AA, Mattos CHPDS, Santos EASD, Neto NRM, Moreira RP, Batella LT, et al. Oral nutritional supplementation in cancer patients who were receiving chemo/chemoradiation therapy: A multicenter, Randomized Phase II Study. Nutrition and Cancer. 2021;**73**(3):442-449. DOI: 10.1080/01635581.2020.1758170

[116] Wu XS, Yousif L, Miles A, Braakhuis A. A comparison of dietary intake and nutritional status between aged care residents consuming texture modified diets with and without oral nutritional supplements. Nutrients. 2022;**14**(3):1-13. DOI: 10.3390/nu14030669

[117] Shune S, Barewal R. Redefining the value of snacks for nursing home residents: Bridging psychosocial and nutritional needs. Geriatric Nursing. 2022;**44**:39-47. DOI: 10.1016/j.gerinurse.2021.12.022

[118] Johnstone AM, Stephen S. Chapter 8—Energy balance: Impact of

physiology and psychology on food choice and eating behavior. In: Marriott BP, Birt DF, Stallings VA, Yates AA, editors. Present Knowledge in Nutrition 8th ed. London: Academic Press: 2020. pp. 143-158. DOI: 10.1016/B978-0-12-818460-8.00008-3

[119] Donini LM. Chapter 2—Control of food intake in aging. In: Raats MM, de Groot LCPGM, van Asselt D, editors. Food for the Aging Population. 2nd ed. Woodhead Publishing; 2017. pp. 25-55. DOI: 10.1016/B978-0-08-100348-0.00002-0

[120] Côté C, Giroux A, Villeneuve-Rhéaume A, Gagnon C, Germain I. Is iddsi an evidence-based framework? A relevant question for the frail older population. Geriatrics (Switzerland). 2020;**5**(4):1-16. DOI: 10.3390/geriatrics5040082

[121] Cichero JA, Altman KW. Definition, prevalence and burden of oropharyngeal dysphagia: A serious problem among older adults worldwide and the impact on prognosis and hospital resources. Nestle Nutrition Institute Workshop Series. 2012;**72**:1-11. DOI: 10.1159/000339974

[122] Maslow AH. A theory of human motivation. Psychological Review. 1943;**50**(4):370-396. DOI: 10.1037/h0054346

[123] Potts R. Introduction to Human Evolution. Smithsonian Institute; 2022 [Website]. Available from: https://humanorigins.si.edu/education/introduction-human-evolution

[124] Ledogar JA, Dechow PC, Wang Q, Gharpure PH, Gordon AD, Baab KL, et al. Human feeding biomechanics: Performance, variation, and functional constraints. PeerJ. 2016;**2016**(7):1-47. DOI: 10.7717/peerj.2242

[125] Le Magnen J. Hunger. In: Problems in the Behavioural Sciences. United States: Cambridge University Press; 1985

[126] Spence C. The tongue map and the spatial modulation of taste perception. Current Opinion in Food Science. 2022;**5**:598-610. DOI: 10.1016/j.crfs.2022.02.004

[127] Ji M, Su X, Su X, Chen Y, Huang W, Zhang J, et al. Identification of novel compounds for human bitter taste receptors. Chemical Biology & Drug Design. 2014;**84**(1):63-74. DOI: 10.1111/cbdd.12293

[128] McMullen MK. Neural transmission from oropharyngeal bitter receptors to the medulla is partially or completely labelled-line. Natural Product Communications. 2016;**11**(8):1201-1204. DOI: 10.1177/1934578x1601100841

[129] Simmen B, Hladik A, Ramasiarisoa PL, Iaconelli S, Hladik CM. Taste discrimination in lemurs and other primates, and the relationships to distribution of plant Allelochemicals in different habitats of Madagascar. In: Publishers KAP, editor. New Directions in Lemur Studies. New York; 1999. pp. 201-209

[130] Lee H, MacPherson LJ, Parada CA, Zuker CS, Ryba NJP. Rewiring the taste system. Nature. 2017;**548**(7667):330-333. DOI: 10.1038/nature23299

[131] Spielman AI, Brand JG. Wiring taste receptor cells to the central gustatory system. Oral Diseases. 2018;**24**(8):1388-1389. DOI: 10.1111/odi.12833

[132] Spector AC, Blonde G, Garcea M, Jiang E. Rewiring the gustatory system: Specificity between nerve and taste bud field is critical for normal salt discrimination. Brain Research. 2010;**1310**:46-57. DOI: 10.1016/j.brainres.2009.11.021

[133] Peng Y, Gillis-Smith S, Jin H, Tränkner D, Ryba NJP, Zuker CS. Sweet and bitter taste in the brain of awake behaving animals. Nature. 2015;**527**(7579):512-515. DOI: 10.1038/nature15763

[134] Cattaneo C, Gargari G, Koirala R, Laureati M, Riso P, Guglielmetti S, et al. New insights into the relationship between taste perception and oral microbiota composition. Scientific Reports. 2019;**9**(1):1-8. DOI: 10.1038/s41598-019-40374-3

[135] Cattaneo C, Riso P, Laureati M, Gargari G, Pagliarini E. Exploring associations between interindividual differences in taste perception, oral microbiota composition, and reported food intake. Nutrients. 2019;**11**(5):1-17. DOI: 10.3390/nu11051167

[136] Esberg A, Haworth S, Hasslöf P, Holgerson PL, Johansson I. Oral microbiota profile associates with sugar intake and taste preference genes. Nutrients. 2020;**12**(3):1-19. DOI: 10.3390/nu12030681

[137] Fluitman KS, van den Broek TJ, Nieuwdorp M, Visser M, Ijzerman RG, Keijser BJF. Associations of the oral microbiota and Candida with taste, smell, appetite and undernutrition in older adults. Scientific Reports. 2021;**11**(1):1-11. DOI: 10.1038/s41598-021-02558-8

[138] Kaur K, Sculley D, Veysey M, Lucock M, Wallace J, Beckett EL. Bitter and sweet taste perception: Relationships to self-reported oral hygiene habits and oral health status in a survey of Australian adults. BMC Oral Health. 2021;**21**(1):1-11. DOI: 10.1186/s12903-021-01910-8

[139] Mozhdehi FJ, Abeywickrema S, Bremer PJ, Peng M. Comparing taste detection thresholds across individuals following vegan, vegetarian, or omnivore diets. Foods. 2021;**10**(11):1-11. DOI: 10.3390/foods10112704

[140] Sedghi L, DiMassa V, Harrington A, Lynch SV, Kapila YL. The oral microbiome: Role of key organisms and complex networks in oral health and disease. Periodontology 2000. 2021;**87**(1):107-131. DOI: 10.1111/prd.12393

[141] Koc H, Vinyard CJ, Essick GK, Foegeding EA. Food oral processing: Conversion of food structure to textural perception. Annual Review of Food Science and Technology. 2013;**4**(1): 237-266. DOI: 10.1146/annurev-food-030212-182637

[142] Foster KD, Grigor JM, Cheong JN, Yoo MJ, Bronlund JE, Morgenstern MP. The role of oral processing in dynamic sensory perception. Journal of Food Science. 2011;**76**(2):R49-R61. DOI: 10.1111/j.1750-3841.2010.02029.x

[143] González R, Montoya I, Cárcel J. The use of electromyography on food texture assessment. Food Science and Technology International. 2001;**7**(6): 461-471. DOI: 10.1106/NRHT-L39D-HY1Y-8RGB

[144] Taniguchi H, Tsukada T, Ootaki S, Yamada Y, Inoue M. Correspondence between food consistency and suprahyoid muscle activity, tongue pressure, and bolus transit times during the oropharyngeal phase of swallowing. Journal of Applied Physiology. 2008;**105**(3):791-799. DOI: 10.1152/japplphysiol.90485.2008

[145] Funami T, Ishihara S, Kohyama K. Use of electromyography in measuring food texture. Food Texture Design and Optimization. Wiley Blackwell; 2014:283-307. 10.1002/9781118765616.ch11

[146] Tournier C, Grass M, Septier C, Bertrand D, Salles C. The impact of mastication, salivation and food bolus formation on salt release during bread consumption. Food & Function. 2014;**5**(11):2969-2980. DOI: 10.1039/c4fo00446a

[147] Mori K, Manda Y, Kitagawa K, Nagatsuka H, Furutera H, Kodama N, et al. Coordination of surface electromyography activity in the

posterior tongue region during mastication of differently textured foods. Journal of Oral Rehabilitation. 2021;**48**(4):403-410. DOI: 10.1111/joor.13135

[148] Matsuo K, Kito N, Ogawa K, Izumi A, Masuda Y. Effects of textured foods on masticatory muscle activity in older adults with oral hypofunction. Journal of Oral Rehabilitation. 2020;**47**(2):180-186. DOI: 10.1111/joor.12901

[149] Steele CM. The blind scientists and the elephant of swallowing: A review of instrumental perspectives on swallowing physiology. Journal of Texture Studies. 2015;**46**(3):122-137. DOI: 10.1111/jtxs.12101

[150] Guo Q. Understanding the oral processing of solid foods: Insights from food structure. Comprehensive Reviews in Food Science and Food Safety. 2021;**20**(3):2941-2967. DOI: 10.1111/1541-4337.12745

[151] Matsuo K, Fujishima I. Textural changes by mastication and proper food texture for patients with oropharyngeal dysphagia. Nutrients. 2020;**12**(6):1-15. DOI: 10.3390/nu12061613

[152] Drake MA. Sensory evaluation. In: McSweeney PLH, McNamara JP, editors. Encyclopedia of Dairy Sciences. 3rd ed. Oxford: Academic Press; 2022. pp. 572-576. DOI: 10.1016/B978-0-12-818766-1.00151-3

[153] Stone H, Bleibaum RN, Thomas HA editors. Sensory Evaluation Practices. 5th ed. London: Academic Press; 2020

[154] Meiselman HL, Schutz HG. History of food acceptance research in the US Army. Appetite. 2003:**40**(3):199-216. DOI: 10.1016/S0195-6663(03)00007-2

[155] Bourne MC. Chapter 1—Texture, viscosity, and food. In: Bourne MC, editor. Food Texture and Viscosity. San Diego: Academic Press; 2012:1-32. DOI: 10.1016/B978-0-12-119060-6.50006-X

[156] Stone H, Bleibaum RN, Thomas HA. Chapter 1—Introduction to sensory evaluation. In: Stone H, Bleibaum RN, Thomas HA, editors. Sensory Evaluation Practices. 4th ed. San Diego: Academic Press; 2012:1-21. DOI: 10.1016/B978-0-12-382086-0.00001-7

[157] Peryam DR, Pilgrim FJ. Hedonic scale method of measuring food preferences. Food Technology. 1957;**11**(Suppl):9-14

[158] Peryam DR, Girardot NJGSHS. Advanced Taste-Test Method. 1998

[159] Wichchukit S, O'Mahony M. The 9-point hedonic and unstructured line hedonic scales: An alternative analysis with more relevant effect sizes for preference. Food Quality and Preference. 2022;**99**:104575. DOI: 10.1016/j.foodqual.2022.104575

[160] Mongi RJ, Gomezulu AD. Descriptive Sensory Analysis, Consumer Preference, and Conjoint Analysis of Beef Sausages Prepared from a Pigeon Pea Protein Binder. SSRN (Social Science Research Network). 2022. Under Review. DOI: 10.2139/ssrn.4047097

[161] Gupta MK, Gonzalez Viejo C, Fuentes S, Torrico DD, Saturno PC, Gras SL, et al. Digital technologies to assess yoghurt quality traits and consumers acceptability. 2022

[162] Vucea V, Keller HH, Morrison JM, Duncan AM, Duizer LM, Carrier N, et al. Nutritional quality of regular and pureed menus in Canadian long term care homes: An analysis of the Making the Most of Mealtimes (M3) project. BMC Nutrition. 2017;**3**(1):1-11. DOI: 10.1186/s40795-017-0198-3

[163] Cichero JAY, Lam P, Steele CM, Hanson B, Chen J, Dantas RO, et al. Development of international terminology and definitions for texture-modified foods and thickened fluids used in dysphagia management: The IDDSI framework. Dysphagia. 2017;**32**(2):293-314. DOI: 10.1007/s00455-016-9758-y

[164] Stahlman LB, Garcia JM, Chambers E, Smit AB, Hoag L, Chambers DH. Perceptual ratings for pureed and molded peaches for individuals with and without impaired swallowing. Dysphagia. 2001;**16**(4):254-262. DOI: 10.1007/s00455-001-0084-6

[165] Sharma M, Kristo E, Corredig M, Duizer L. Effect of hydrocolloid type on texture of pureed carrots: Rheological and sensory measures. Food Hydrocolloids. 2017;**63**:478-487. DOI: 10.1016/j.foodhyd.2016.09.040

[166] Rothenberg E, Ekman S, Bülow M, Möller K, Svantesson J, Wendin K. Texture-modified meat and carrot products for elderly people with dysphagia: Preference in relation to health and oral status. Scandinavian Journal of Food and Nutrition. 2007;**51**(4):141-147. DOI: 10.1080/17482970701760675

[167] Wendin K, Ekman S, Bülow M, Ekberg O, Johansson D, Rothenberg E, et al. Objective and quantitative definitions of modified food textures based on sensory and rheological methodology. Food & Nutrition Research. 2010;**54**:1-11. DOI: 10.3402/fnr.v54i0.5134

[168] Martínez O, Vicente MS, De Vega MC, Salmerón J. Sensory perception and flow properties of dysphagia thickening formulas with different composition. Food Hydrocolloids. 2019;**90**:508-514. DOI: 10.1016/j.foodhyd.2018.12.045

[169] Ross AIV, Tyler P, Borgognone MG, Eriksen BM. Relationships between shear rheology and sensory attributes of hydrocolloid-thickened fluids designed to compensate for impairments in oral manipulation and swallowing. Journal of Food Engineering. 2019;**263**:123-131. DOI: 10.1016/j.jfoodeng.2019.05.040

[170] Cichero JAY, Steele C, Duivestein J, Clavé P, Chen J, Kayashita J, et al. The need for international terminology and definitions for texture-modified foods and thickened liquids used in dysphagia management: Foundations of a global initiative. Current Physical Medicine and Rehabilitation Reports. 2013;**1**(4):280-291. DOI: 10.1007/s40141-013-0024-z

[171] Felt P. The National Dysphagia Diet Project: The science and practice. Nutrition in Clinical Practice. 1999;**14**(5):S60-SS5. DOI: 10.1177/088453369901400513

[172] Mills RH. Rheology overview: Control of liquid viscosities in dysphagia management. 1999;**14**(5S):S52-SS6. DOI: 10.1177/0884533699014005S11

[173] Tymchuck D. Textural property considerations of food for dysphagia. 1999;**14**(5S):S57-SS9. DOI: 10.1177/0884533699014005S12

[174] Côté C, Germain I, Dufresne T, Gagnon C. Comparison of two methods to categorize thickened liquids for dysphagia management in a clinical care setting context: The Bostwick consistometer and the IDDSI flow test. Are we talking about the same concept? Journal of Texture Studies. 2019;**50**(2):95-103. DOI: 10.1111/jtxs.12377

[175] Sherman P. Food Texture and Rheology. London: Academic Press; 1979

[176] Gallegos C, Turcanu M, Assegehegn G, Brito-de la Fuente E. Rheological issues on oropharyngeal dysphagia. Dysphagia. 2021:1-28. DOI: 10.1007/s00455-021-10337-w

[177] Raheem D, Carrascosa C, Ramos F, Saraiva A, Raposo A. Texture-modified food for dysphagic patients: A comprehensive review. International Journal of Environmental Research and Public Health. 2021;18(10):1-24. DOI: 10.3390/ijerph18105125

[178] Szczesniak AS. Classification of textural characteristics. Journal of Food Science. 1963;**28**(4):385-389. DOI: 10.1111/j.1365-2621.1963.tb00215.x

[179] Szczesniak AS, Brandt MA, Friedman HH. Development of standard rating scales for mechanical parameters of texture and correlation between the objective and the sensory methods of texture evaluation. Journal of Food Science. 1963;**28**(4):397-403. DOI: 10.1111/j.1365-2621.1963.tb00217.x

[180] van der Stelt AJ, Mehring P, Corbier C, van Eijnatten EJM, Withers C. A "mouthfeel wheel" terminology for communicating the mouthfeel attributes of medical nutrition products (MNP). Food Quality and Preference. 2020;**80**:1-11. DOI: 10.1016/j.foodqual.2019.103822

[181] Deeks J, Verreault MF, Cheung W. Canadian nutrient file (CNF): Update on Canadian food composition activities. Journal of Food Composition and Analysis. 2017;**64**:43-47. DOI: 10.1016/j.jfca.2017.04.009

[182] Bodner-Montville J, Ahuja JKC, Ingwersen LA, Haggerty ES, Enns CW, Perloff BP. USDA Food and Nutrient Database for Dietary Studies: Released on the web. Journal of Food Composition and Analysis. 2006;**19**(Suppl):S100-S1S7. DOI: 10.1016/j.jfca.2006.02.002

[183] Charrondiere UR, Vignat J, Møller A, Ireland J, Becker W, Church S, et al. The European Nutrient Database (ENDB) for nutritional epidemiology. Journal of Food Composition and Analysis. 2002;**15**(4):435-451. DOI: 10.1006/jfca.2002.1089

[184] Watanabe T. Food composition tables of Japan and the nutrient table/database. Journal of Nutritional Science and Vitaminology (Tokyo). 2015;**61**(Suppl):S25-S27. DOI: 10.3177/jnsv.61.S25